D1605250

CHINESE *TUINA* THERAPY

Wang Fu

FOREIGN LANGUAGES PRESS   BEIJING

First Edition 1994

Translated by Fang Tingyu and Zhang Kai

ISBN 7-119-01674-1

© Foreign Languages Press, Beijing 1994
Published by Foreign Languages Press
24 Baiwanzhuang Road, Beijing 100037, China

Printed by Beijing Foreign Languages Printing House
19 Chegongzhuang Xilu, Beijing 100044, China

Distributed by China International Book Trading Corporation
35 Chegongzhuang Xilu, Beijing 100044, China
P.O. Box 399, Beijing, China

Printed in the People's Republic of China

PREFACE

Tuina is a simple therapy which uses neither medicine nor medical devices, but uses various massage techniques to stimulate the body to regulate the bodily functions and eliminate pathogenic factors. Originating in China *tuina* therapy has now been adopted in many countries around the world. In China a wealth of experience in *tuina* therapy has been accumulated and doctors have developed a system of techniques which has helped cure many illnesses. To introduce this therapy around the world, I was asked by the Foreign Languages Press to supplement and revise the book, *Popular Tuina Therapy,* published by the People's Hygiene Publishing House, and expand it into a new book, *Chinese Tuina Therapy*, which includes thirty *tuina* manipulations and twenty-nine therapies for common diseases.

I hope readers will find this book helpful and learn from it.

Author

CHAPTER ONE
GENERAL INTRODUCTION

I. HISTORY OF *TUINA* THERAPY

Chinese *tuina* therapy has a long history. As early as 500,000 or 600,000 years ago Peking Man learned how to use fire. Primitive man was able to make objects out of bones and crude stoneware. The "Upper Cave Man" living 100,000 years ago could make bone objects and stoneware with holes. People went out in groups to seek food and lived in shelters built on trees to escape attacks from wild animals. Every day they had to climb up and jump from the trees dozens of times. They fought fierce wild animals in collecting food and hunting. Physical injury and strains were unavoidable. In addition, aching and numb limbs and gastro-intestinal disorders due to affliction of cold or summer heat, and a raw and cold diet occurred frequently. People stroked the hurt part of the body to relieve the pain. Repeated strokes helped people to understand how to relieve pain and so primitive massage began to take shape.

The primitive *tuina* therapy was quite simple without specific manipulations based on systematic knowledge. Alongside the evolution of man and accumulation of knowledge, masseurs as healers came into being. Masseurs were experienced people who were frequently visited.

Legend has it that from c. 26th century B.C. to c. 22nd century on 21st century B.C. there were masseurs such as Jiu Daiji. Huang Di was an ancient emperor who enjoyed high prestige, and Qi Bo was his private physician who also taught him medicine. Yu Fu, also serving as Huang Di's private physician and Qi Bo were of the same generation. *The Yellow Emperor's Canon of Medicine*, the oldest and most comprehensive work on medicine still extant, appeared around 300 B.C., in the style of questions and answers on problems of medicine between Qi Bo and Huang Di. A passage in the book says: "In the Central Plains of China it is damp and many inhabitants suffer from soreness, pain and numbness of the limbs and joints due to pathogenic wind, cold and dampness, for which *daoyin*[1] and massage are the best therapies."

It indicates that even in ancient China *tuina* was an important medical approach. It is stated in the *Records of the Historian* by Sima Qian (around 145 or 135 B.C.—?), a historian in the Western Han Dynasty (206 B.C.-24 A.D), that there

---

[1] A kind of treatment by pressing and rubbing the limbs by oneself to take away pain and stiffness from the muscles and joints.

3

had been a practitioner named Yu Fu who treated patients with *bian* stones (a kind of needle made out of stone used in external treatment), *daoyin* and massage instead of herbal decoctions.

Tuina was used in the Western Zhou Dynasty (c. 11th century B.C.-771 B.C.) and the Warring States Period (475 B.C.-221 B.C.). Bian Que (about 500 B.C.), an early noted physician, rescued a dying crown prince of the Zhao State with acupuncture and *tuina* therapy. His skill at bringing a dying man back to life won admiration. It was widely spoken about and is listed in the *Records of the Historian*, becoming the first written successful case record of *tuina* therapy.

The discipline of *tuina* therapy developed in the Qin and Han dynasties (221 B.C.-220 A.D) and *tuina* therapy played a significant role in medical treatment. In this period monographs on *tuina* therapy appeared in the *History of the Han Dynasty* which says that there was a book entitled *Ten Volumes of Tuina Therapy by Huang Di and Qi Bo*, but the book was unfortunately lost. The Wei, Jin and Southern and Northern dynasties (220-550) witnessed new advances in *tuina* therapy. Ge Hong (281-341), a physician in the Jin Dynasty (265-420), wrote a book named *Nei Pian, Bao Pu Zi,*[1] in which a volume of *Canon of the Tuina Therapy* and ten volumes of the *Classic of Daoyin* were mentioned. He said: "Pressing and rubbing the affected part of the body cures the complaints." Hua Tuo (?-208), famous surgeon in the Three Kingdoms (220-280), and his pupils were good at massage and *daoyin*. Knowledge of massage and *daoyin* was recorded in the *General Treatise on the Causes and Symptoms of Diseases* by Chao Yuanfang (550-630) in the Sui Dynasty (581-618), indicating their extensive use. A *tuina* department was set up in the Imperial Health Administration in the Tang Dynasty (618-907). The *New Tang Dynasty History* presented in a series of biographies points out in the Imperial Health Administration there were "two court academicians of massage and four masseurs. They treated fractures, contusions and strains. It suggests that masseurs at that time also treated traumas. It is described in the *Decrees and Regulations of the Tang Dynasty* that there were fifty-six masseurs and fifteen massage pupils in the Imperial Health Administration." From the above we know that there was a massage department with a considerable number of professionals with four academic titles, i.e. court academicians, high-rank masseurs, low-rank masseurs and pupils, showing the importance of the *tuina* therapy and that there was a training program for masseurs in the Tang Dynasty. The manipulations of *tuina* therapy had advanced too. For example, in the *Valuable Prescriptions*, written by Sun Simiao (581-682), a renowned physician skilled at massage, illustrated the eighteen manipulations of massage developed by Lao Zi (an ancient philosopher). Sun was known for his medical skills, even by later generations and he lived to be over hundred. A massage tool, the bamboo rod created in the Tang Dynasty was used as an aid to alleviate the workload of masseurs, since patients were too numerous to be treated.

---

1 This is a book recording the experience of the Chinese people in pharmaceutical chemistry.

Emphasizing the Confucian ethical code rather than technical knowledge, the rulers of the Song Dynasty (960-1279) dismantled the Massage Department from the Imperial Health Administration. But it was still quite popular among the masses. Pang Anshi was a celebrated physician and a great massage specialist in the Song Dynasty. One woman had difficult labour and after seven days the baby had still not been delivered. Pang was called in to help. He first warmed the lower back of the woman with hot water, then he massaged her whole body. Afterwards a baby boy was delivered. This is an example showing how a difficult labour was helped by massage. Volume 4 of the *Imperial Encyclopedia of Medicine* compiled by the Imperial Health Administration in the Song Dynasty says: "Pressing and rubbing one's hand on the body is called massage. Pressing is only done by hands whereas rubbing can be conducted with medicinal herbs," which shows that rubbing medication on the body was also done at that time. *Tuina* therapy did not advance in the Song Dynasty and the Yuan Dynasty (1271-1368). But it developed again in the Ming Dynasty (1368-1644), especially for infants. Heavy pressure is not suitable for infants because of their delicate constitutions. As *tuina* therapy developed, it gradually became the main form of massage. In the Ming Dynasty special works on *tuina* therapy appeared, e.g., *Points of Infant Tuina Therapy* by Zhou Zifang, *Infant Tuina Methods and Points Observed* by Gong Yunlin, and Chen's *A Classic of Infant Massage*.

The Qing Dynasty (1644-1911) witnessed more publications on *tuina* therapy. They were: *A General Discription of Tuina Therapy* by Xiong Yingxiong, *Secret of Infant Tuina Therapy* by Luo Rulong, *Records of Infant Tuina Therapy* by Qian Huaicun, *Important Skills of Massage* by Zhang Zhenjun and *A Shortcut for Tuina Therapy* by Ma Yushu. *Important Skills of Massage* is an illustrated enlarged edition of the *Secret of Tuina Therapy*, in which palpation of the chest and abdomen and point location were added to the four diagnostic methods—inspection, auscultation interrogation and palpitation.

The Golden Mirror of Medicine, an encyclopedia of traditional Chinese medicine, is one of the best treatises of general medicine written by a staff of 80, headed by Wu Qian in compliance with an imperial order. "The Treatise of Bone-Setting Methods" in the book states: "It is advisable to treat bone fractures associated with stagnation of *qi*, blood stasis, swelling and pain due to injuries with massage. The meridians are pressed to make *qi* flow *smoothly*, and the swollen part is rubbed to remove blood stasis." The book includes the eight treating methods—feeling, joining, raising, lifting, pressing, rubbing, pushing, and pulling, among which over four methods are concerned with *tuina* therapy. It proves that traumology was developed on the basis of *tuina* therapy. *Tuina* was among the thirteen medical branches at the Imperial Health Administration in the Ming and Qing dynasties. Acupuncture and *tuina* were discriminated against only in the later stage of the Qing Dynasty. The rulers thought they were "insignificant in the medical system," "did not appeal to refined tastes" and "were improper to be included in the therapies for the imperial family." Since then acupuncture and *tuina* were dismissed from the Imperial Health Administration. During the regime of the Kuomintang (1927-1949), the government, following in the footsteps of the rulers of the Qing Dynasty, discriminated against acupuncture and *tuina* therapy, which were on the verge of dying out. Since the founding of the People's Republic of China in 1949, *tuina* therapy was accepted again, as well as traditional Chinese medicine and both have made great progress. *Tuina* therapy hospitals and departments in general hospitals have been set up in provincial, municipal and autonomous region levels since 1956. *Tuina* schools and training courses have started to train *tuina* practitioners. Many *tuina* practitioners have disseminated their clinical experience and published some papers and books. Furthermore, books on traditional massage have been written by doctors of the Western medical system learning traditional Chinese medicine. They have contributed to the inheritance and development of *tuina* therapy.

II. THE BASIC THEORY OF *TUINA* THERAPY

1. Origin of *Tuina* Therapy

Practice has shown that *tuina* therapy cure ailments, but it is quite difficult to see what is behind it. Research is providing a better understanding of *tuina* therapy. Many talented scholars who are doing research with modern scientific techniques conclude that Western medicine has been very successful in researching anatomy, but some disorders that were not cured by Western drugs and surgical operations have been solved by *tuina* therapy.

2. The Theoretical Foundation of *Tuina* Therapy

Tuina therapy brings about changes in the body through stimulations induced by manipulations and movement of the body and limbs without using drugs or medical apparatus. Experiments show that *tuina* therapy may decrease or increase the number of white cells in different cases. The nutrients in the body can be adjusted and the harmful agents eliminated with *tuina* therapy by strengthening of the phagocytes, which destroy bacteria, thus complaints can be relieved or healed. Muscular pain is alleviated or eliminated when *tuina* therapy is applied, not only because the abnormal muscular condition is healed, but also because there is a change in the acid-base scale in the muscles.

Traditional Chinese medicine holds that nature is comprised of two opposing, yet uniting forces *yin* and *yang* which are also reflected in nature. This is the concept of integrity viewed by traditional Chinese medicine. People vary individually. Under the same climatic conditions some are attacked by illnesses and some are not, simply because of the individual body resistance. The viewpoint of diversification in traditional medical theory is the starting point of understanding physiology and pathology. It is stated in the "Treatise on the Correspondence

Between the Man and the Universe" in *Plain Questions* that, *"Yin* and *yang* are the way of the heaven and earth, the great outlines of everything, the parents of all changes, the origin of birth and death, and the source of all mysteries." In terms of anatomy, the upper part of the body is *yang* and the lower part *yin*; the exterior is *yang* and the interior *yin*; the back is *yang* and the abdomen *yin;* the *fu*-organs are *yang* and the *zang*-organs *yin*. *Yin* and *yang* depend on each other for existence. Without *yin*, there would be no *yang*. Without *yang*, there would be no *yin*. Neither can exist in isolation. The coordination of the *yin-yang* aspects ensures the body's normal development. When an excess or deficiency of *yin* or *yang* appears, then the body is transformed from its healthy state into a diseased condition. For example, *yang* is impaired by an excess of *yin* and vice versa. A deficiency of *yin* leads to interior heat, while a deficiency of *yang* lead to exterior cold. The function of *tuina* therapy is to regulate *yin* and *yang* to maintain their dynamic balance, so as to eliminate the root cause of a disease. The basic theory of traditional Chinese medicine determines the treating principle of the *tuina* therapy which uses neither medications nor needles.

In addition, a normal, physiological relationship should exist between the five *zang* organs (heart, liver, spleen, lung and kidney) and the six *fu* organs (gallbladder, stomach, small intestine, large intestine, triple *jiao* and urinary bladder). An abnormal, disturbing, pathological relationship can also exist between them. Normal and abnormal bodily functions are connected with normal and abnormal changes of nature. A deep understanding of pathological disorders plays an important role in *tuina* therapy. Not only awareness of internal disorders is dependent on the theories of traditional Chinese medicine, but treatment of limb complaints is also guided by them. For example, "when the lung and heart are involved in a pathogenic invasion, pathogenic *qi* lingers in both elbows; when the liver is involved, it lingers in both axillae; when the spleen is involved, it lingers in both groins; when the kidney is involved, it stays in both popliteal fossae." Other theories such as "the spleen nourishes the muscles," "the lung is associated with the skin surface," "the condition of the liver determines the conditions of the sinews," are also helpful to the therapeutics in analysis and diagnosis of the disease cause.

What is *qi*? According to Chinese medical theory, *qi* is the fundamental substance constituting the universe, and all phenomena are produced by the changes and movement of *qi*. *Qi* is the essential substance of the human body and maintains its vital activities. Zhang Jingyue, a famous practitioner in the Ming Dynasty (1562-1639), pointed out, *"Qi* is the source of human life." There is no explanation of *qi* by modern medicine because anatomy is a scientific study of the body based on dissection of the corpse, and of course no *qi* can be seen in a dead body. The existence of *qi* has been proven by modern scientific techniques and the theory plays an important role in *tuina* therapy. Activating the smooth flow of *qi* and blood is the aim of the *tuina* therapy. "Pain is usually caused by blood insufficiency due to invasion of pathogenic cold into the meridians of the back. Massage applied to the diseased site brings a warm sensation, which alleviates the pain" ("Treatise on abrupt Pains" in *Plain Questions*). The above explains the harm of pathogenic cold and the function of massage.

The meridian theory is another important guide in *tuina* therapy because it determines pathology, diagnosis and treating principles.

The meridians, run longitudinally within the body, while the collaterals, which are branches of the meridians, run horizontally from the meridians. They are collectively termed *jingluo* (meridians and collaterals) in traditional Chinese medicine. This system of meridians and collaterals includes the twelve regular meridians (three *yin* meridians of the hand, three *yang* meridians of the hand, three *yin* meridians of the foot and three *yang* meridians of the foot), the eight extraordinary meridians (Du Meridian, Ren Meridian, Chong Meridian, Dai Meridian, Yinwei Meridian, Yangwei Meridian, Yinqiao Meridian and Yangqiao Meridian), and the fifteen collaterals. Besides, there are twelve divergent meridians, the twelve muscle regions and cutaneous regions, tertiary collaterals and superficial collaterals. Among them, the twelve regular meridians and the Ren and Du Meridians in total are called the fourteen meridians. The nomenclature of the twelve meridians is based which category they belong to, for example, since the Hand-Taiyin meridians belong to *yin*, they are called the Lung Meridians of Hand-Taiyin. The nomenclature of the meridians according to the name of the *zang-fu* organs stresses their correlations with the given *zang* and *fu* organs. The diversity of hand and foot meridians indicates their chief location. Furthermore, they also have *yin* and *yang* aspects. First, traditional Chinese medicine considers that the five *zang* organs and pericardium pertain to *yin*, while the six *fu* organs to *yang*. Then the meridians that pertain to the *zang* organs are *yin* meridians and those pertaining to the *fu* organs are *yang* meridians. Points on the given meridian can be used to treat disorders of the related individual organ. Second, those travelling along the medial aspect of the limbs, chest and abdomen are *yin* meridians, while those travelling along the lateral aspect of the limbs, back and head are *yang* meridians.

The extraordinary meridians, eight in total, have specific functions. The importance of the Ren and Du Meridians is similar to the twelve regular meridians and the other six are less important in comparison.

Each of the fourteen meridians has a collateral and together with the Great Collateral of the Spleen, there are fifteen collaterals. The course along which they travel is parallel with that of the related meridians.

The tertiary collaterals are known as the subdivided small branches of the meridians or capillaries. The twelve divergent meridians are those going out from the regular meridians and running in the deeper part of the body. The twelve muscle regions of the twelve regular meridians are those parts distributed in the exterior of the four limbs, trunk, head and face (including some in the chest and abdomen), connecting only with the muscles rather than the internal organs. The twelve cutaneous regions are superficial capillaries in which meridian *qi* travels and they are closely related with the superficial collaterals.

The meridians reflect the concept of integrity in traditional Chinese medical theory. The system of meridians and collaterals is a crisscross network, internally connected with the five *zang* and six *fu* organs and externally with the four limbs and six *fu* organs and externally with the four limbs and the superficial tissues, skeleton, five sense organs, and nine body orifices. Their action is to regulate the function of different organs, connect the external with internal organs, thus making the body an organic whole and maintaining a dynamic balance between various parts of the body.

It is pointed out in the "Treatise on the Original Organs" from *Mireculous Pivot* that "The meridians and collaterals transport blood and *qi* to adjust *yin* and *yang*, nourish tendons and bones, and improve joint function." The meridians and collaterals are passages for the circulation of *qi* and blood, which bring nutrients to the tissues and organs, providing the necessities for the smooth functioning of the body and maintaining a relative equilibrium of normal activities. All of this is known as the vital function of meridians, the failure of which results in invasion of pathogenic factors into the body. For this reason it can be well said that nutrients are brought to the whole body through the function of the meridians and the invasion of the pathogenic factors is also through the meridians too. Only by completely understanding the theory of meridians can one be aware of the body's self-adjusting capacity and use *tuina* therapy flexibly. In addition to the fundamental knowledge of meridians and points, therapists have to know the function of some specific points—the Back-Shu points, Front-Mu points and Yuan-Primary points.

The Back-Shu points include twelve points, i.e., Feishu (B 13), Jueyinshu (B 14), Xinshu (B 15), Ganshu (B 18), Danshu (B 19), Pishu (B 20), Weishu (B 21) Sanjiaoshu (B 22), Shenshu (B 23), Dachangshu (B 25), Xiaochangshu (B 27) and Pangguangshu (B 28). The ancient Chinese considered these points to be the places where *qi* of the respective *zang-fu* organs is infused and that they are the points selected when the *zang-fu* organs are in trouble.

Front-Mu points include twelve points, i.e., Zhongfu (L 17), Tianshu (S 25), Zhongwan (R 12), Zhangmen (Liv 13), Juque (Ren 14), Guanyuan (Ren 4), Zhongji (Ren 3), Jinmen (B 63), Tanzhong (Ren 17), Shimen (Ren 5), Riyue (G 24) and Qimen (Liv. 14). The Chinese ancients held that the Front-Mu points are those where *qi* of the respective *zang-fu* organs is infused. They play an important role in the diagnosis and treatment of the disorders of the internal organs (but in many cases, they are used together with the Back-Shu points.)

Yuan-Primary points include the following: Taiyuan (L 9), Hegu (LI 4), Chongyang (S 42), Taibai (Sp 3), Shenmen (H 7), Wangu (G 12), Jingu (B 64), Taixi (K 3), Daling (P 70), Yangchi (TE 4), Qiuxu (G 40) and Taichong (Liv 3). They are located in the vicinity of the wrist and ankle and are good for internal disorders.

Influential points include the following eight points. They are Zhangmen (Liv 13), Zhongwan (Ren 12), Yanglingquan (G 34), Jueque (G 39), Geshu (B 17), Dazhu (B 11), Taiyuan (L 9) and Tanzhong (Ren 17). They are used to treat disorders of the *zang* organs, *fu* organs, *qi*, blood, tendons, vessels, bones and marrow.

Luo-Connecting points are the following fifteen points, i.e., Pianli (LI 6), Lieque (L 7), Gongsun (Sp 4), Tongli (H 5), Zhizheng(SI 7), Fenglong (S 10), Jiuwei (Ren 15), Dazhong (K 4), Feiyang (B 58), Waiguan (TE 5), Neiguan (P 6), Ligou (Liv 5), Guangming (G 37), Changqiang (Du 1) and Dabao (Sp 21). They are used to dredge the meridians for the smooth flow of *qi* and blood in combination with other points on the fourteen meridians.

The above knowledge can help us to integrate the local condition with the whole body in the application of massage, especially in the treatment of internal disorders, the Back-Shu and Front-Mu points are really helpful. For example, Tanzhong (Ren 17), an influential point of *qi* is selected as a secondary point to treat impeded flow of *qi*, or Geshu (B 17), an influential point of blood, is used to treat blood disorders. It is easier to understand the indications and functions of other points when we have the knowledge of these points.

3.Commonly-Used Meridians, Points and Their Indications

See the table below.

Location and Indications of Commonly-Used Meridians and Points

Meridian	Point	Location	Indications
Lung Meridian of Hand-Taiyin	Zhongfu (L 1)	Laterosuperior to the sternum at the lateral side of the 1st intercostal space	Cough, asthma, pain in the chest, shoulder and back
	Chize (L 5)	On the cubital crease, on the radial side of the tendon of the m. biceps brachii	Cough, asthma, fullness of the chest, spasmodic pain of the elbow and arm
	Lieque (L 7)	Superior to the styloid process of the radius, 1.5 *cun* above the transverse crease of the wrist	Sore throat, migraine, wrist and elbow pain, and tenosynovitis
Large Intestine Meridian of Hand-Yangming	Shangyang (LI 1)	On the radial side of the index finger, about 0.1 *cun* posterior to the corner of the nail	Toothache, and loss of consciousness due to apoplexy
	Hegu (LI 4)	On the dorsum of the hand, between the 1st and 2nd metacarpal bones	Toothache, headache, common cold, pain of the arm, and apoplexy
	Quchi (LI 11)	When the elbow is flexed, the point is in the depression at the lateral end of the transverse cubital crease.	Elbow pain, and hemiplegia

	Shousanli (LI 1)	2 *cun* below Quchi (LI 5)	Toothache, nasal obstruction, headache, pain in the shoulder and arm, and hemiplegia
	Jianyu (LI 15)	Anterior-interior to the acromion, on the upper portion of m. deltoideus	Pain in the the shoulder and arm, motor impairment of the upper limbs, and hemiplegia
	Yingxiang (LI 20)	In the nasolabial groove, at the level of the midpoint of the lateral border of the ala nasi	Nasal obstruction, and facial paralysis
Triple *Jiao* Meridian of Hand-Shaoyang	Tianjin (SJ 10)	When the elbow is flexed, the point is in the depression about 1 *cun* superior to the olecranon.	Pain in the shoulder and arm, and migraine
	Sizhukong (SJ 23)	In the depression at the lateral end of the eyebrow	Migraine, facial paralysis, squint, and eye trouble
Pericardium Meridian of Hand-Jueyin	Quze(P 3)	On the transverse cubital crease, at the ulnar side of the tendon of the m. biceps brachii	Angina pectoris, pain in the elbow and arm, irritability, and palpitation
	Neiguan (P 6)	2 *cun* above the transverse crease of the wrist, between the tendons of the m. palmaris longus and the m. flexor radialis	Tachycardia, bradycardia, angina pectoris, arrhythmia, hypertension, stomachache, pain in the hypochondriac region, and hysteria
Heart Meridian of Hand-Shaoyin	Jiquan (H 1)	When the upper arm is abducted, the point is in the centre of the axilla.	Pain in the elbow, arm and costal region, and inflammation around the shoulder joint
	Shaohai (H 3)	When the elbow is fixed into a right angle, the point is in the depression between the medial end of the transverse cubital crease and the medial epicondyle of the humerus.	Cardiac pain and numbness of the hand and arm
Small Meridian of Hand-Taiyang	Tianzhong (SI 11)	In the infrascapular fossa, at the junction of the upper and middle third of the distance between the lower border of the scapular spine and the inferior angle of the scapula	Pain in the scapular region, and motor impairment of the shoulder
	Jianwaishu (SI 14)	3 *cun* lateral to the lower border of the spinous process of the 1st thoracic vertebra	Pain and rigidity of the neck, pain and cold sensation in the back, and cervical spondylopathy
Stomach Meridian of Foot-Yangming	Chengqi (S 1)	With the eyes looking straight forward, the point is directly below the pupil, between the eyeball and the infraorbital ridge.	Twitching of eyelids, and blurring of vision
	Dicang (S 4)	0.4 *cun* away from the corner of the mouth, on the line of the pupil	Facial paralysis and twitching of the lips

	Jiache (S 6)	One finger-breadth anterior and superior to the lower angle of the mandible where the m. masseter attaches at the prominence of the muscle when the teeth are clenched	Toothache, deviation of the mouth and eye, and locked jaw
	Xiaguan (S 7)	At the lower border of the zygomatic arch, in the depression anterior to the condyloid process of the mandible	Toothache, deviation of the mouth and eye, and locked jaw
	Touwei (S 8)	0.5 *cun* within the anterior hairline at the corner of the forehead	Headache, and eye pain
	Liangmen (S 21)	4 *cun* above the umbilicus, 2 *cun* lateral to Zhongwan (Ren 12)	Gastric pain, abdominal distension, loose stools, vomiting, and prolapse of the rectum
	Tianshu (S 25)	2 *cun* lateral to the centre of the umbilicus	Diarrhea, constipation, and pain around the umbilicus
	Yinshi (S 33)	When the knee is flexed, the point is 3 *cun* above the laterosuperior border of the patella.	Numbness, soreness and motor impairment of the knee, and lower limbs
	Zusanli (S 36)	3 *cun* below Dubi (S 35), one finger breadth from the anterior crest of the tibia, in m. tibialis anterior	Gastric pain, abdominal pain, diarrhea, hypertension, paralysis, knee pain, and general debility
	Jiexi (S 41)	On the dorsum of the foot, at the midpoint of the transverse crease of the ankle joint, in the depression between the tendons of the m. extensor digitorum longus and the hallucis longus	Headache, and pain in the ankle joint
Bladder Meridian of Foot-Taiyang	Jingming (B 1)	0.1 *cun* superior to the inner canthus	Redness, swelling and pain of the eye, lacrimation, and myopia
	Zanzhu (B 2)	On the medial extremity of the eyebrow	Frontal headache, dizziness, facial paralysis, pain in the supraorbital region, and prosopalgia
	Dazhui (B 11)	1.5 *cun* lateral to Taodao (Du 13), at the level of the lower border of the spinous process of the first thoracic vertebra	Common cold, cough, headache, pain in the scapular region and neck rigidity
	Fengmen (B 12)	1.5 *cun* lateral to the Du Meridian, at the level of the lower border of the spinous process of the 2nd thoracic vertebra	Headache, cough, nasal obstruction, and neck rigidity
	Feishu (B 13)	1.5 *cun* lateral to Shenzhu (Du 12), at the level of the lower border of the spinous process of the 3rd thoracic vertebra	Cough, asthma, fullness of the chest, and pain in the back

Xinshu (B 15)	1.5 *cun* lateral to Shendao (Du 11), at the level of the lower border of the spinous process of the 5th thoracic vertebra	Angina pectoris, arrhythmia, bradycardia, palpitation, and loss of memory
Geshu (B 17)	1.5 *cun* lateral to Zhiyang (Du 9), at the level of the lower border of the spinous process of the 7th thoracic vertebra	Anemia, escape of blood, afternoon fever, and esophagismus
Ganshu (B 17)	1.5 *cun* lateral to Jinguo (Du 8), at the lower border of the spinous process of the 9th thoracic vertebra	Chronic diseases of the liver and gallbladder, pain in the hypochondriac region, backache, and eye complaints
Danshu (B 19)	1.5 *cun* lateral to Zhongshu (Du 7), at the level of the lower border of the spinous process of the 10th thoracic vertebra	Chronic diseases of the liver and gallbladder, dizziness, backache, pain in the hypochondriac region, and bitter taste in the mouth
Pishu (B 20)	1.5 *cun* lateral to Jizhong (Du 6), at the level of the lower border of the spinous process of the 11th thoracic vertebra	Gastric pain, edema, abdominal distension, diarrhea, and diabetes
Weishu (B 21)	1.5 *cun* lateral to the Du Meridian, at the level of the lower border of the spinous process of the 12th thoracic verbetra	Gastric pain, gastroptosis, abdominal pain, backache, and chronic hepatitis
Sanjiaoshu (B 22)	1.5 *cun* lateral to Xuanshu (Du 5), at the level of the lower border of the spinous process of the 1st lumbar vertebra	Indigestion, dysentery, edema, enuresis, and backache
Shenshu (B 23)	1.5 *cun* lateral to Mingmen (Du 4), at the level of the lower border of the spinous process of the 2nd lumbar vertebra	Pain in the lower back and legs, nephritis, hemiplegia, enlargement of the liver, nocturnal emission, impotence, shortness of breath, deafness, and enuresis
Dachangshu (B 25)	1.5 *cun* lateral to Yaoyangguan (Du 3), at the level of the lower border of the spinous process of the 4th lumbar vertebra	Acute and prolonged lower back pain, sciatica, constipation, abdominal distension, borborygmus, and diarrhea
Xiaochangshu (B 27)	1.5 *cun* lateral to the Du Meridian, at the level of the 1st posterior sacral foramen	Abdominal pain, enteritis, pelvic inflammation, morbid leukorrhea, enuresis, nocturnal emission, and lower back pain
Pangguangshu (B 28)	1.5 *cun* lateral to the Du Meridian, at the level of the 2nd posterior sacral foramen	Pain in the lower back, constipation, and enuresis
Ciliao (B 32)	In the second posterior sacral foramen	Lower back pain, muscular atrophy of the lower limbs, irregular menstruation, and dysuria

	Chengfu (B 36)	In the middle of the transverse gluteal fold	Pain in the lower back and gluteal region, sciatica, and paralysis of the lower limbs
	Yimen (B 37)	6 *cun* below Chengfu (B 36)	Acute pain in the lower back, paralysis of the lower limbs, and sciatica
	Weizhong (B 40)	Midpoint of the transverse crease of the popliteal fossa	Lower back pain, complaints of the knee joints, motor impairment of the lower limbs, and muscular atrophy
	Gaohuangshu (B 43)	3 *cun* lateral to the Du Meridian, at the level of the lower border of the spinous process of the 4th thoracic vertebra, on the spinal border of the scapula	Pain and cold sensation in the back, debility, neurasthenia, and nocturnal emission
	Zhaohai (K 6)	In the depression of the lower border of the medial malleolus, or 1 *cun* below the medial malleolus	Sore throat, and constipation
Gallblandder Meridian of Foot-Shaoyang	Tongziliao (G 1)	0.5 *cun* lateral to the outer canthus, in the depression on the lateral side of the orbit	Headache, pain of the eyes, facial paralysis, and myopia
	Yangbai (G 14)	On the forehead, 1 cun directly above the midpoint of the eyebrow	Toothache, facial paralysis, and prosopalgia
	Fengchi (G 20)	In the depression between the upper portion of the m. sternocleidomastoideus and the m. trapezius, on the same level with Fengfu (Du 16)	Common cold, headache, insomnia, hypertension, glaucoma, and optic atrophy
	Jianjing (G 21)	Midway between Dazhui (Du 14) and the acromion, at the highest point of the shoulder	Pain in the shoulder and back, mastitis, and inflammation around the shoulder joint
	Jingmen (G 25)	On the lateral side of the abdomen, on the lower border of the free end of the 12th rib	Pain in the lumbar hypochondriac and spleen regions, and abdominal distension
	Zhishi (B 52)	3 *cun* lateral to Mingmen (Du 4), at the level of the lower border of the spinous process of the 2nd lumbar vertebra	Nocturnal emission, impotence, asthma, and poor functioning of the spleen and stomach
Kidney Meridian of Foot-Shaoyin (K 1)	Kunlun (B 60)	In the depression between the external malleolus and tendo calcaneus	Pain of the heel and lower back and legs
	Shenmai (B 62)	In the depression directly below the external malleolus	Motor impairment and pain in the lower limbs, epilepsy and lower back and neck pain
	Jinmen (B 63)	Anterior and inferior to Shenmai (B 62), in the depression, lateral to the cuboid bone	Motor impairment and pain in the lower limbs, epilepsy and lower back and neck pain

	Yongguan (K 1)	On the sole, in the depression, plantar flexion of the foot, approximately at the juncture of the anterior third and posterior two thirds of the sole	Headache, dizziness, hypertension and pain in the head and neck
	Huantiao (G 30)	At the junction of the lateral 1/3 and medial 2/3 of the distance between the greater trochanter and the hiatus of the sacrum	Pain in the lumbar region and thigh, sciatica, and hemiplegia
	Fengshi (G 31)	On the midline of the lateral aspect of the thigh, 7 *cun* above the transverse popliteal crease	Pain in the lumbar region and thigh, "Bi" syndrome, and general itching
	Yanglingquan (G 34)	In the depression anterior and inferior to the head of the fibula	Hypochondriac pain, sciatica and lateral numbness of the lower limbs
Liver Meridian of Foot-Jueyin	Dadun (Liv 1)	On the lateral side of the dorsum of the terminal phalanx of the great toe, between the lateral corner of the nail and the interphalangeal joint	Hernia, vaginal pain, prolapse of the uterus, and pain in the testis
	Xingjian (Liv 2)	On the dorsum of the foot between the 1st and 2nd toe	Headache, spasm of the facial muscle, pain in the testis, and glaucoma
	Zhangmen (Liv 13)	On the lateral side of the abdomen, below the free end of the 11th floating rib	Hypochondriac pain, enlargement of the spleen, and indigestion
	Qimen (Liv 14)	Directly below the nipple, in the 6th intercostal space	Hypochondriac pain, and mastitis
Ren Meridian	Huiyin (Ren 1)	Between the anus and the root of the scrotum	Irregular menstruation, vaginitis, and nocturnal emission
	Zhongji (Ren 3)	On the midline of the abdomen, 4 *cun* below the umbilicus	Irregular menstruation, prolapse of uterus, vaginal itching, and frequency of urination
	Guanyuan (Ren 4)	On the midline of the adbomen, 3 *cun* below the umbilicus	Lower back pain, diabetes, enteritis, cystitis, and enuresis
	Qihai (Ren 6)	On the midline of the abdomen, 1.5 *cun* below the umbilicus	Abdominal and lumbar pain, dysmenorrhea, and upward attack of liver *qi*
	Jianli (Ren 11)	On the midline of the abdomen, 3 *cun* above the umbilicus	Gastric pain, abdominal distension, poor appetite, edema, and vomiting
	Zhongwan (Ren 12)	On the middle line of the abdomen, 4 *cun* above the umbilicus	Gastric pain, hiccup, abdominal distension, and diarrhea
	Tanzhong (Ren 17)	On the anterior midline, level with the 4th intercostal space midway between the nipple	Angina pectoris, fullness in the chest, mastitis, and insufficient lactation

gular menstruation, annexitis, mastitis, and climacteric syndrome.

(4) Pediatric disorders: Baby night cry, vomiting of milk, whooping cough, malnutrition, dysentery, watery diarrhea, bedwetting, acute and chronic convulsion, five kinds of retardation (in standing, walking, growth of hair, tooth eruption and the faculty of speech), sequela of polio, and prolapse of the rectum.

(5) ENT disorders: Red eyes, mild myopia, stye, tinnitus and nosebleed.

2. Contraindications, Precautions and Commonly-Used Points

(1) Contraindications:
   a. Acute infectious diseases
   b. Locality of tumours
   c. Ulcerating dermatosis
   d. Burns, and scalds
   e. Various infections, suppurative cases, and tuberculous arthritis
   f. Severe heart disease, and liver conditions
   g. Severe mental disorders
   h. Diseases occurring during menstruation and pregnancy (especially those in the abdomen where *tuina* therapy should not be applied)
   i. Gastric and duodenal perforation
   j. Elderly patients who are critically ill
   k. Cases which haven't been treated before (such as bone fracture, and dislocation of the cervical vertebra)

(2) Precautions:

The hands of the masseur must be clean, and the fingernails kept short. The hands should be kept warm in winter and talcum powder is used in massage to prevent the skin from injury. The masseur should be wholly absorbed and the *tuina* therapy must not be applied to patients immediately after overeating and drinking alcohol or to those who have done sports consuming a great deal of strength or on those who are in a rage. Fifteen treatments usually make a course. A long course may decrease the effects. Several days' rest is advisable between two courses.

(3) Commonly-used points (Figs. 1-1/9)

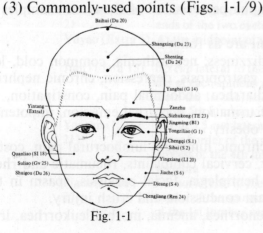

Fig. 1-1

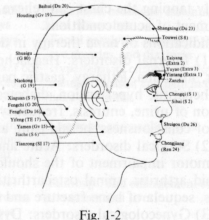

Fig. 1-2

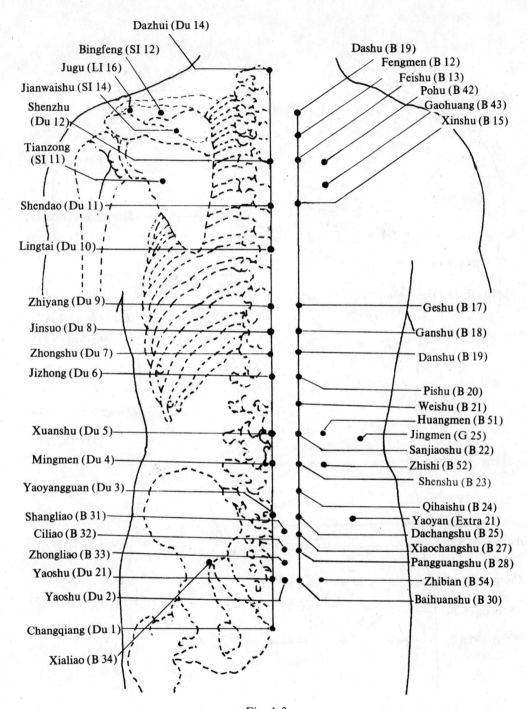

Fig. 1-3

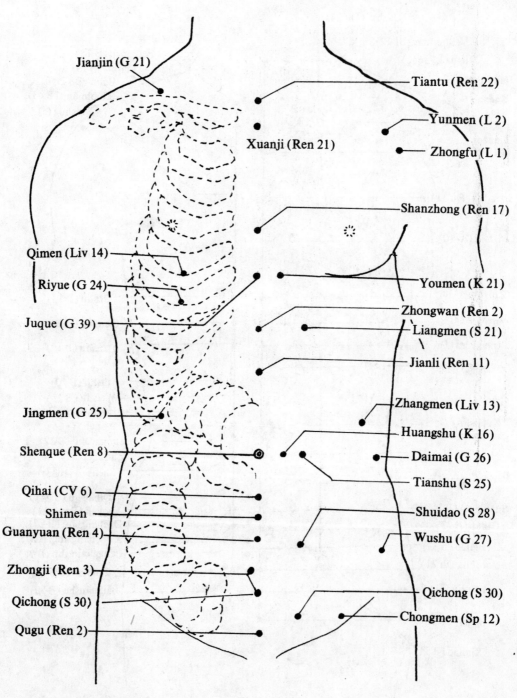

Jianjin (G 21)
Tiantu (Ren 22)
Yunmen (L 2)
Xuanji (Ren 21)
Zhongfu (L 1)
Shanzhong (Ren 17)
Qimen (Liv 14)
Riyue (G 24)
Youmen (K 21)
Zhongwan (Ren 2)
Liangmen (S 21)
Juque (G 39)
Jianli (Ren 11)
Zhangmen (Liv 13)
Jingmen (G 25)
Huangshu (K 16)
Shenque (Ren 8)
Daimai (G 26)
Tianshu (S 25)
Qihai (CV 6)
Shuidao (S 28)
Shimen
Wushu (G 27)
Guanyuan (Ren 4)
Zhongji (Ren 3)
Qichong (S 30)
Qichong (S 30)
Chongmen (Sp 12)
Qugu (Ren 2)

Fig. 1-4

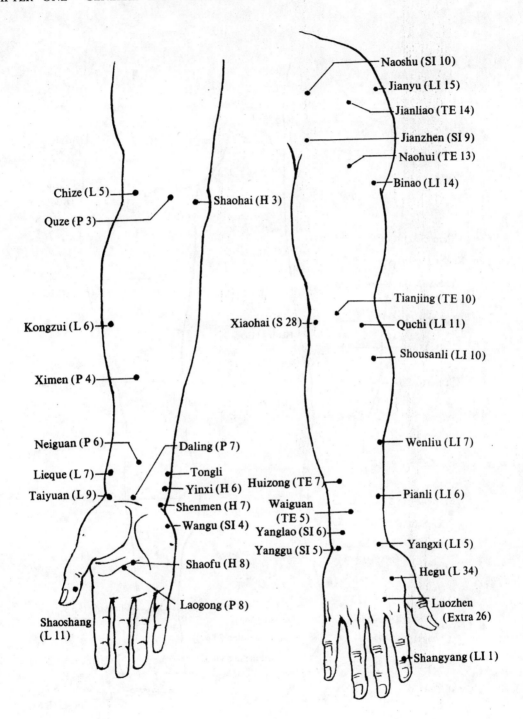

Chize (L 5)
Quze (P 3)
Shaohai (H 3)
Naoshu (SI 10)
Jianyu (LI 15)
Jianliao (TE 14)
Jianzhen (SI 9)
Naohui (TE 13)
Binao (LI 14)
Kongzui (L 6)
Xiaohai (S 28)
Tianjing (TE 10)
Quchi (LI 11)
Shousanli (LI 10)
Ximen (P 4)
Neiguan (P 6)
Daling (P 7)
Tongli
Lieque (L 7)
Yinxi (H 6)
Huizong (TE 7)
Wenliu (LI 7)
Taiyuan (L 9)
Shenmen (H 7)
Waiguan (TE 5)
Pianli (LI 6)
Wangu (SI 4)
Yanglao (SI 6)
Yanggu (SI 5)
Yangxi (LI 5)
Shaofu (H 8)
Hegu (L 34)
Laogong (P 8)
Luozhen (Extra 26)
Shaoshang (L 11)
Shangyang (LI 1)

Fig. 1-5   Fig. 1-6

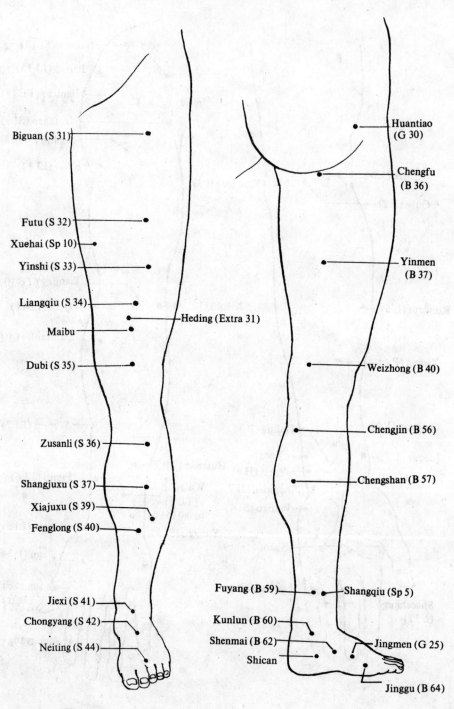

Biguan (S 31)

Futu (S 32)

Xuehai (Sp 10)

Yinshi (S 33)

Liangqiu (S 34)

Maibu

Heding (Extra 31)

Dubi (S 35)

Zusanli (S 36)

Shangjuxu (S 37)

Xiajuxu (S 39)

Fenglong (S 40)

Jiexi (S 41)

Chongyang (S 42)

Neiting (S 44)

Fig. 1-7

Huantiao (G 30)

Chengfu (B 36)

Yinmen (B 37)

Weizhong (B 40)

Chengjin (B 56)

Chengshan (B 57)

Fuyang (B 59)

Shangqiu (Sp 5)

Kunlun (B 60)

Shenmai (B 62)

Jingmen (G 25)

Shican

Jinggu (B 64)

Fig. 1-8

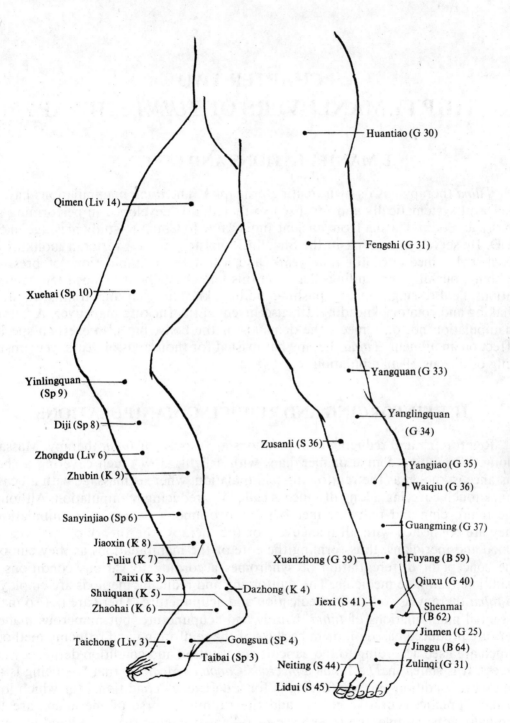

Fig. 1-9

CHAPTER TWO
THIRTY MANEUVERS OF *TUINA* THERAPY

I. MANIPULATIONS AND EFFECTS

Tuina therapy has its own treating principles. The *tuina* manipulations have to be learnt systematically and practised so that skill is developed in performing the massage. Bodhi-dharma from ancient India came to China to study massage in 507 A.D. He served as a monk in the Shaolin Monastery with a verteran monk as his teacher. He meditated for nine years, and learnt the manipulations of pressing, rubbing, pushing and pulling. Based on this knowledge he developed ten manipulations, i.e. Pressing, rubbing, pushing, pulling, kneading, jerking, rolling, twisting, shaking and rotatory kneading. He also invented the flicking maneuver. A helpful manipulation not only meets the demands of the body, but also exerts a specific effect on an ailment. *Tuina* therapy has existed for thousands of years, yet consists only of dozens of manipulations.

II. REINFORCING AND REDUCING MANIPULATIONS

Reinforcing and reducing manipulations are aspects of *tuina* therapy. Massage along the running course of meridians with a light, slow touch covering a short distance is known as the reinforcing manipulation, whereas massage with a heavy, quick touch covering a long distance is called the reducing manipulation. Although the reinforcing and reducing methods are two among dozens of manipulations, they are connected with all maneuvers of the therapy, the theory of *yin-yang, qi*, blood and meridians, thus forming the core of the manipulations as they embody the concept of differentiation of syndromes according to various conditions in traditional Chinese medicine. The reinforcing and reducing methods are employed in *tuina* therapy as well as in medication and acupuncture. There are not so many essential manipulations of *tuina* therapy and acupuncture, but numerous maneuvers are produced based on them because of the reinforcing and reducing methods, which are used according to the patients constitution and condition-deficiency and excess. It is stated in *The Yellow Emperor's Canon of Medicine* that "reducing is for an excess condition and reinforcing is for a deficiency condition," for which long medical practice, curative effects and the running course of meridians are the grounds. For example, the three *yang* meridians originate from the hand to head, heavy massage applied along the course is called reinforcing and heavy massage against the course is known as reducing. The three *yin* meridians travel from the chest to the hand. Massage in a downward direction along the meridians is called reinforcing, otherwise it is called reducing. The Du Meridian runs from the coccygeal to head. Heavy massage applied in an upward direction is called reinforcing and vice versa. The Ren Meridian goes upward from the midline of the lower abdomen. Massage in an upward direction is called reinforcing and otherwise it is called reducing. For a beginner it is important to know the course of the meridians and the commonly-used points, on the basis of which varieties of manipulations can be used. Massage from the right to the left in males is called reinforcing, from the left to right reducing, whereas that from the left to right in females is called reinforcing, from the right to left reducing. These are known as the left-right reinforcing and reducing methods. A light, quick, soft touch of short duration is called the reinforcing method and a heavy, deep touch of a long duration is called the reducing method. These are the light-heavy reinforcing and reducing methods. Upward massage from the umbilicus is called reinforcing and downward massage from the umbilicus is called reducing. Massage along and against the running course of meridians with heavy and light touches is called even reinforcing and reducing method. The reinforcing and reducing methods are not necessarily applied to mild cases. Without it satisfactory effects can also be obtained. The masseur often uses these methods unconsciously, because in practice heavy and light, quick and slow touches are alternately applied and this is either the reinforcing or reducing method. Only for severe and complicated conditions or for prolonged chronic cases with marked symptoms are the reinforcing and reducing methods used, so as to accurately and effectively cure a disease. Carelessness could in fact injure a patient. Needless to say, experienced *tuina* therapyists are able to apply the reinforcing and reducing manipulations skillfully, so they have to have the knowledge of the reinforcing and reducing manipulation necessary for some cases.

III. THIRTY MANEUVERS OF *TUINA* THERAPY

1. Stroking Maneuver (See Fig. 2-1)

This is done by passing the hands gently over a part of the body or the whole body from upward to downward or vice versa starting from the end of the limbs three to five times.

Main points observed: The working palms should be slightly bent and not completely touch the body, only with the pads of the fingers and the palmaris. Stroking lightly stimulates the nerves of the skin, producing a very comfortable feeling.

Functions: This technique is used to excite the peripheral nerves, dilate capillaries, disperse pain of the central nerves and relax the deep muscles.

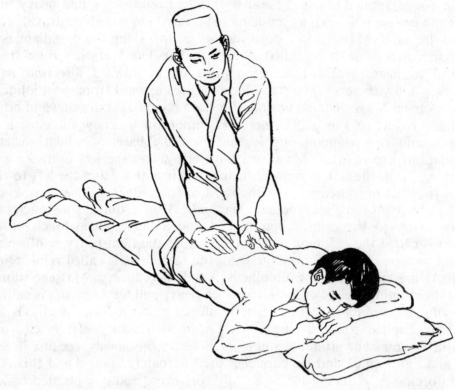

Fig. 2-1

　　This is a maneuver used before massage or in the intervals of massage with various techniques. Seeing simple, it is an important technique. Anyone who practises *Taijiquan* knows the importance of the preparatory posture. A good preparatory posture can help one enter a quiescent state, relax himself and regulate the *qi* so that it descends to *Dantian*, which is considered the basis of the practice of *Taijiquan*. Without any preparation immediate practice of *Taijiquan* only brings a confused condition and failure to perform the movements properly. It is the same with the preparatory maneuver in *tuina* therapy. It helps the patient enter a quiescent state, to relax his muscles and promote smooth blood circulation. That is why this maneuver is discussed first because the success of the massage depends on it. Adults and the elderly prefer this maneuver, but some oversensitive people don't like because it creates an intolerable itching feeling in them. In these cases heavier stroking is done by using the whole palm to massage the body, or a horizontal pushing maneuver is used. Therefore, the stroking maneuver can never be overlooked and it serves as an adjustment between various manipulations. After heavier manipulations have been applied, a few strokes are given to regulate and make the body relax. It is similar to music, in which a nice harmony will be produced only when there is a coordination of different tones. In terms of massage,

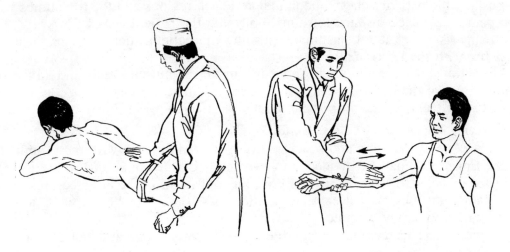

Fig. 2-2   Fig. 2-3

if there are solely heavy or light manipulations, *tuina* therapy will not be effective.

2. Pushing Maneuver (See Figs. 2-2/3)

This technique may be divided into three methods, i.e., (1). Horizontal Pushing

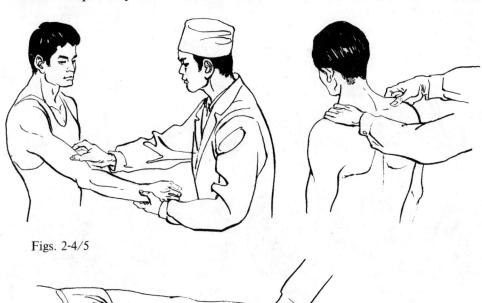

Figs. 2-4/5

Fig. 2-6

—pushing the patient's chest, abdominal and back regions and the four limbs with the palms. (2). Back upward Pushing —pushing the patient's back upwardly with the palmaris. (3). Lateral Pushing —pushing the patient's depressed parts of the vertebra with the lateral palm.

Functions: This technique is applied to make the muscles relax and adjust the temperature of the skin by the action of the deep muscles to produce a comfortable and relaxed feeling. Talcum powder should be used to avoid injury of the skin.

3. Grasping Maneuver (See Figs. 2-4/6)

It is done by grasping and squeezing the affected muscles with the thumb and index fingers. It may be divided into two methods: grasping and squeezing the affected muscles for some time and grasping and twisting the affected muscles.

Main points observed: Heavy stimulation may be done or heavy, moderate and light stimulation may be done.

Functions: This techuique is used to remove *qi* stagnation and blood stasis, and to stop pain.

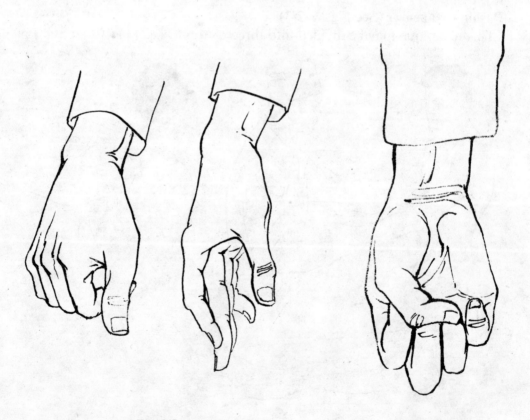

Fig. 2-7   Fig. 2-8

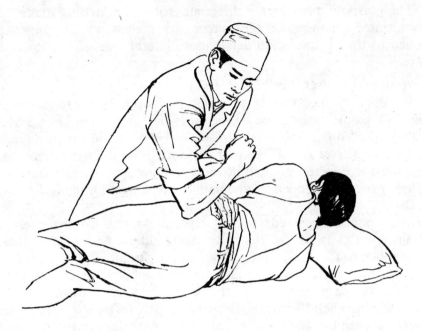

Fig. 2-9

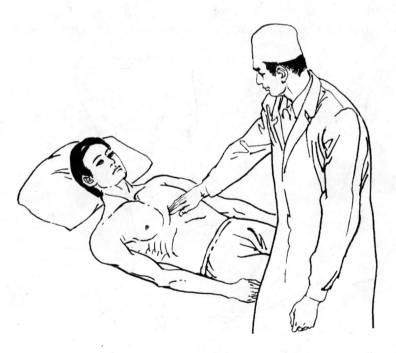

Fig. 2-10

The grasping maneuver is different from the pinching maneuver. The force is concentrated on the pads of fingers rather than on the fingertip. It is usually applied to the armpit, shoulder tendon, lateral side of the lower back, nape and limbs.

4. Pressing Maneuver (See Figs. 2-7/11)

It is done by the doctor by pressing the acupoints and tenderness with the finger (Fig. 2-7), palms (one or one on the other, Fig. 2-11), fist (Fig. 2-8) and elbow (Fig. 2-9) for some time. The chief difference between the touching maneuver and the pressing maneuver is that the former exerts a light force whereas the latter exerts a heavier force. The weighing down technique may be included in this technique, i.e. heavy pressing is doen by one palm, two palms or one on the other over a larger area.

Main points observed: Light pressing is done on the chest and abdominal regions and to any part of the body of the elderly and infants. Heavier pressing is only applied to the back, lower back and hip of adults. But the force only transmits to the deep muscles and the affected part which creates a sore and distending sensation in the patient. When the palm is pressed down, the force is gradually increased and when it reaches the affected part (after the appearance of a sore and distending feeling), the force is decreased. When doing the maneuver, never exert pressure suddenly because doing so may injure the patient or injure the fingers and hands of the doctor himself.

Functions: This technique is used to promote the smooth flow of *qi* in the meridians, stop pain through cold elimination or anesthesia or strengthen diges-

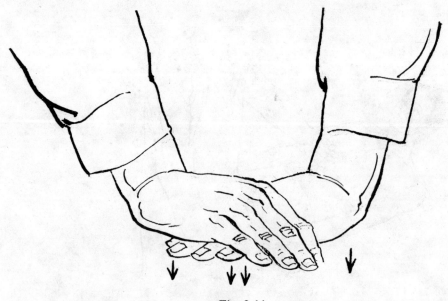

Fig. 2-11

tion. It can also regulate the nervous function, improve blood circulation, increase the supply of oxygen and nutrients and remove stagnation in the lymph nodes.

5. Palm-rubbing Maneuver (See Fig. 2-12)

It is done by a repeated rubbing of the acupoints or tender spots in the chest and abdomen of the patient with the pads of the thumb, index and middle fingers and the thenar. Both hands conduct the maneuver with even force and rhythm.

Main points observed: Light and gentle rubbing is done with a slow rhythm which will create a comfortable sensation at the affected part. The speed of the rubbing is dependent on the condition. It is usually applied to the swelling contracture and cirrhotic parts, or to the place where stagnancy is present due to cold.

Functions: It is applied to regulate the *qi* flow and the function of the stomach, invigorate blood circulation, eliminate inflammation and fever, disperse cold to

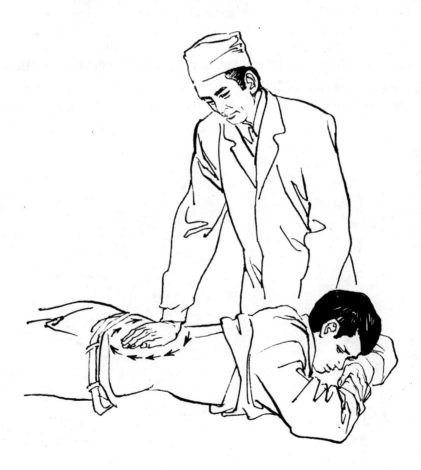

Fig. 2-12

relieve pain, and activate the blood circulation to eliminate blood stasis. It can also help raise the temperature of the skin, improve the function of the sebaceous and sweat glands, remove aging cells, speed up the reflux of the capillary blood and lymph, regulate the central nerves and the function of the peripheral nerves. It may also have an analgesic action and help to relieve pain. It is especially good for infants.

6. Rotatory Kneading Maneuver (See Fig. 2-13)

This is a manipulation similar to the rubbing maneuver, done with the pads of fingers and thenar to the affected area in a rotary movement or an up-and-down movement. When using this technique, the finger always touches the skin and moves the subcutaneous tissue in a circle, e.g., rotatory kneading of the temple. Light force is usually exerted and sometimes heavier force is gradually given.

Main points observed: The same as that of the rubbing maneuver.

Functions: It is used to eliminate swelling, muscular contracture, thecal cyst, strains of the hand or foot, indigestion, headache and constipation.

The rotatory kneading maneuver is usually long and repeatedly conducted at a part to remove or alleviate swelling. Clockwise or counterclockwise kneading is done as you please. Heavier rotatory kneading is only applied to the thecal cyst.

7. Twisting Maneuver (See Fig. 2-14)

This technique is done by twisting the affected part repeatedly and slowly with

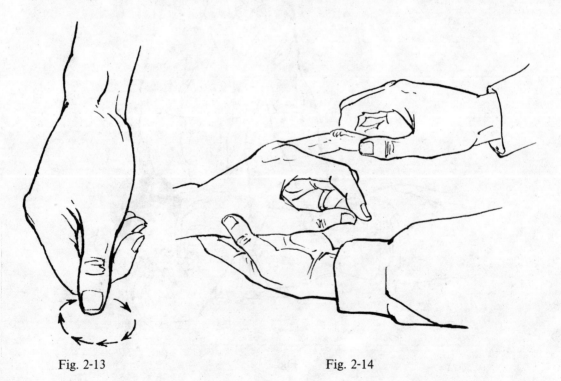

Fig. 2-13   Fig. 2-14

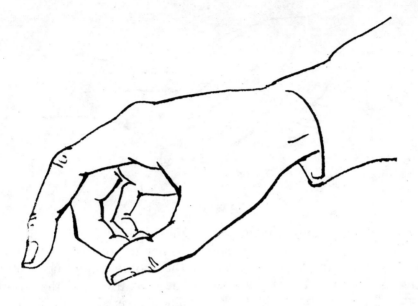

Fig. 2-15

the thumb and index fingers.

    Main points observed: This technique is usually applied to the fingers and toes, because they have more minor joints, and other tecnniques can not be easily used. It is especially helpful for alleviating problems of the finger endings. The vessels of the finger joint are very fine and tend to be blocked. The twisting maneuver may dredge the vessels of the minor joints.

8. Flicking Maneuver (See Fig. 2-15)

    It is done as it is illustrated in Fig. 2-15. The middle or index fingertip is placed under the pad of the thumb. When the thumb gives a resistance and the middle finger exerts a force outwardly, the middle finger is strongly flicked and hits the affected part. It is usually applied to the minor joints of fingers, commonly known as "flicking the vessels of the joints." An experienced doctor can concentrate his strength on the finger to achieve a very good effect. But clinical practice tells us that it is not necessary to use this technique strongly because finger joints are sensitive to pain and the affected part often cannot tolerate the finger force on it. A slight flick is enough to vibrate the *qi* and blood in the body and remove stagnancy in the collaterals, thus "a local breakthrough brings about the total openness of the meridians. For example, a woman of about 40 with rheumatoid athritis came for treatment. She had a sharp pain and contracture in the first joint

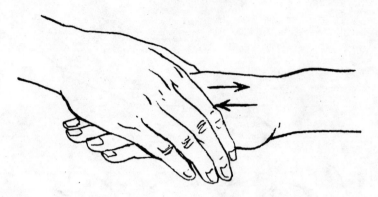

Fig. 2-16

of the thumb and motor impairment of the right shoulder, from which she suffered greatly. There had not been any response to other treatments. After the twisting maneuver was done, the pain ceased, but the motor impairment of the right shoulder remained. Then the flicking technique was used and the motor impairmant improved. Furthermore, the flicking maneuver is also helpful in numbness of fingers.

9. Finger-rubbing Maneuver (See Fig. 2-16)

This technique is done by slight rubbing of the fingers, dorsum of the hand, face and nose with closed fingers. Rubbing is usually done using three fingers, i.e. a finger of the patient is slightly rubbed by three closed up fingers from the nail

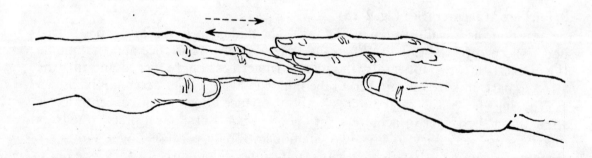

Fig. 2-17

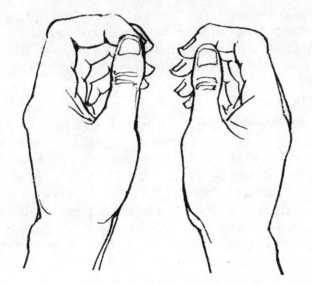

Fig. 2-18

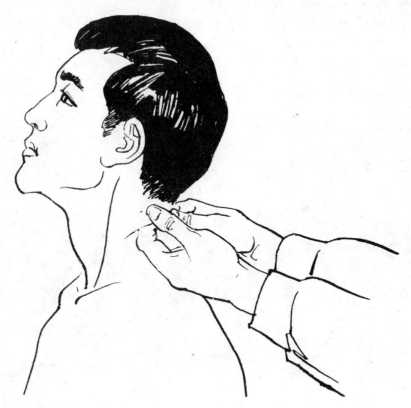

Fig. 2-19

end to the end of a finger as shown in Fig. 2-17. It is good for the reflux of blood in the fingertip, stops pain and removes stasis to help the opened collaterals work smoothly. If there is congestive apex of nose this technique may promote blood reflux. The back of the hand and foot, face and knee joint are often gently rubbed by the palm to finish the *tuina* therapy.

10. Pick-up Maneuver (See Figs. 2-18/19)

This technique is done using the thumb and index finger to take hold of the skin and lift it. This technique is usually applied to a limited area, such as the face, or a man's genitals. If it is used to relieve distending pain, a gentle force is applied with a long duration and crush injury should be avoided. If it is used to remove gelosis and numbness (muscular contracture), forceful picking is applied to the extent that the patient does not feel marked pain. The effect is obtained through slow manipulation. It is especially good for acute mastitis with gentle and frequent manipulations. For gelosis in the face and facial paralysis, the force of pulling is gradually increased without the consciousness of the patient. The action of the picking-up maneuver is similar to that of the pulling maneuver, but it is usually applied to the part where the latter cannot be used.

11. Pinching Maneuver (See Fig. 2-20)

With this technique the doctor presses appropriate acupoints, such as Ren-

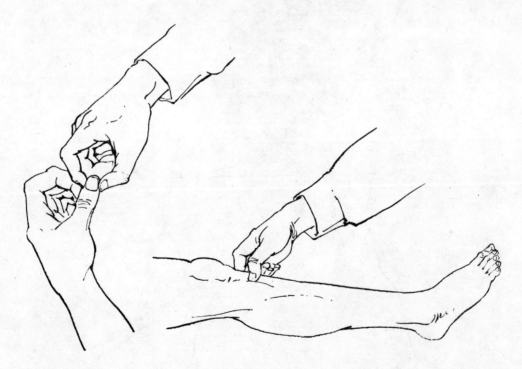

Fig. 2-20

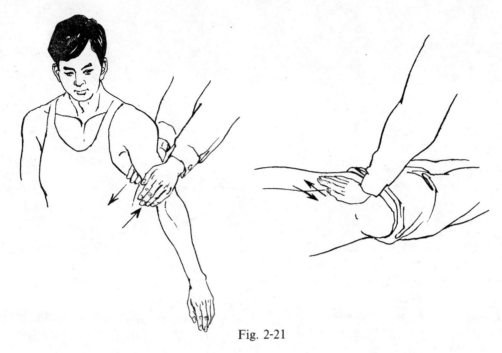

Fig. 2-21

zhong (Du 26), Chengjiang (Ren 24), Sifeng (Extra 29) and Baxie (Extra 28) with his finger nails.

Main points observed: Moderate force must be exerted and the nail must not cut the skin.

Functions: It is used to treat shock, loss of consciousness, dispel pathogenic factors, and harmonize meridians to kill pain.

12. Rubbing Maneuver (See Fig. 2-21)

This technique is done by the doctor by pressing hard on the patient's limbs or lower back with his palms with rotatory movements, or by rubbing the arm with his two palms alternately.

Main points observed: Even force is exerted by the doctor.

Functions: It is used to improve the temperature of the skin, promote *qi* and blood circulation, remove stagnancy to kill pain and reinforce the function of the kidney, urinary bladder and small and large intestines.

13. Rolling Maneuver (See Figs. 2-22/23)

This technique is done by the doctor by using the ulnar side of the dorsum of the hand and the middle, ring and little fingers to compress the patient's body surface by continuously rolling the hand right and left by the wrist force, usually applied to the thigh, shoulder, back, lower back, arms and neck.

Main points observed: The little and ring fingers are slightly bent. A loose fist is formed and the affected part is compressed by the medial fist first, then the fist

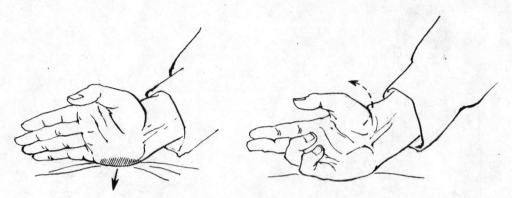

Fig. 2-22/23

is turned outward and the thenar begins to compress the affected part. The movement is repeated several times. It is a very frequently used technique for a larger area of the body surface. It can help sustain the effects of other techniques, therefore, it is often used in the later stage of treatment.

Functions: It is used to dredge the meridians and activate *qi* and blood circulation, remove blood stasis and alleviate pain. It is also helpful to the function of a muscle group.

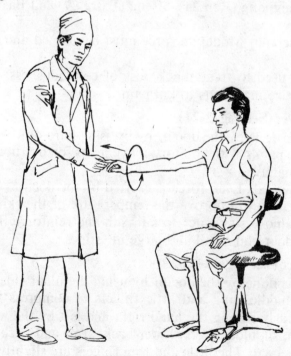

Fig. 2-24

14. Shaking Maneuver (See Fig. 2-24)

This technique is done by the doctor by holding the middle finger of the patient and shaking upwards, to and fro gently and pulling it downward. Then, when all the muscles are relaxed, the doctor pulls the finger suddenly.

Functions: It is used to promote the body's *qi* and blood circulation because the Pericardium Meridian of Hand-Jueyin runs to the middle finger. When there is a smooth flow of *qi* and blood in the Pericardium Meridian, the free flow of *qi* and blood in the whole body is achieved. Jerking of the middle finger is equal to traction of the long head of the biceps brachii muscle, and as a result, contracture, pain and numbness are relieved.

15. Gripping Maneuver (See Fig. 2-25)

To do this technique the doctor bends his index and middle fingers with the thumb on the bent index finger, to be placed between the affected finger and

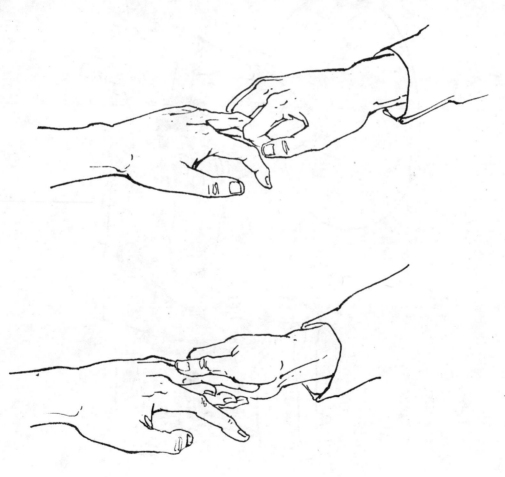

Fig. 2-25

forcefully to smooth out. Sometimes four fingers (except the thumb) put together and smooth out the affected finger, but the action is not so good as the former method.

Main points observed: The affected finger should not gripped too tightly and too loosely, and when the smooth-out maneuver is being applied, there is a pressure on the blood vessels, muscles and bone of the affected finger. Too tight gripping affects the movements of the working fingers or the skin may be injured. If the pain and numbness cannot be alleviated, the affected finger should also be smoothed out laterally.

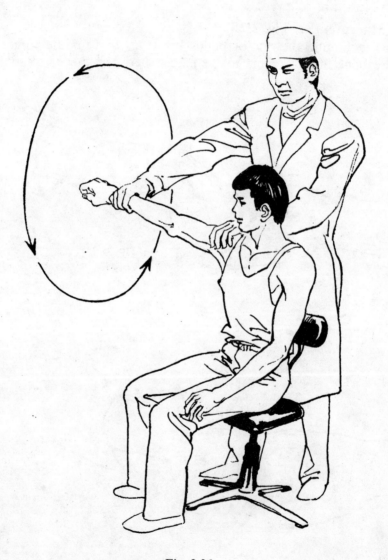

Fig. 2-26

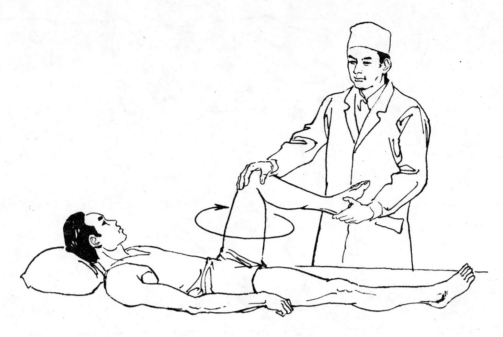

Fig. 2-27

Functions: It is used not only for relieving pain, but also for activating the smooth flow of *qi* and blood in the body, because it can strengthen the peripheral circulation and stimulate the peripheral nerves.

16. Rotating Maneuver (See Figs. 2-26/27)

The doctor moves a joint in a circulatory fashion, e.g., at the head, arm, hip, trunk, wrist and foot.

Main points observed: This technique is applied to a joint where there is obvious motor impairment. The aim of the technique is to restore the joint function, therefore the extent of rotation is dependent on the condition and necessity. The function of the affected joint is gradually restored and a new injury could appear if the treatment is applied with undue haste. The rotation should not produce any sharp pain in the patient.

Functions: This technique is used to relieve motor impairment of a joint and improve *qi* and blood circulation. When the muscles and ligaments around the joint are pulled, their function can be restored.

17. Tapping Maneuver (See Fig. 2-28)

The body is tapped with the palm, usually applied to a larger area of the surface and some other parts, e.g. the shoulder, back, lower back, hip, limbs cubital fossa, and back of the knee. How much force is exerted depends on the condition.

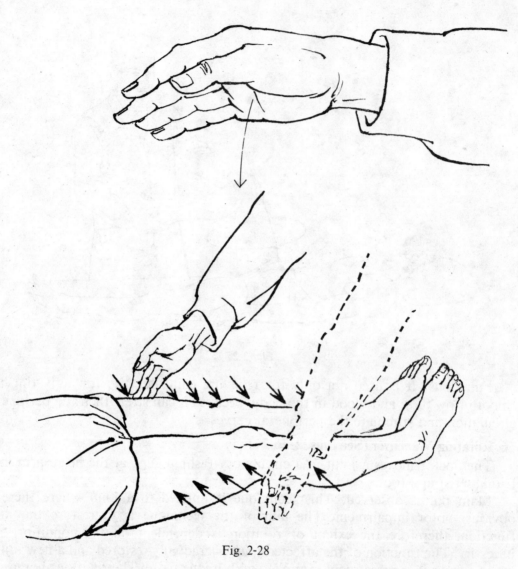

Fig. 2-28

Functions: This technique is used to remove stasis, activate blood and *qi* circulation, dredge meridians, kill pain and numbness and regulate nervous functions. In his "*Eighteen Maneuvers of Tuina Therapy*, Chen Yuqing, a late *tuina* therapist from Hunan Province, pointed out that the tapping maneuver might increase the number of white cells, treat heatstroke and invigorate the tendons. The tapping maneuver has a unique function. For example, if the sole of the foot is hurt by a nail, the sole should be strongly tapped to bring out blood in purple after the nail is removed. In this way, the wound will heal up by itself when no medication is given. This is my clinical experience in treating such a wound.

Doctor Chen Yuqing advised that the cubital fossa and the back of knee until presence of purpura should be tapped for heatstroke with symptoms of sharp abdominal pain, vomiting and diarrhea. With this treatment mild cases can be cured and severe cases alleviated. Several tappings are given with force progressively increasing. This technique can enhance the function of other manipulations, so it can be applied alone or in combination with others.

18. Stretching Maneuver (See Fig. 2-29)

The doctor quickly lifts the muscle on the back with his thumb and the second part of the index finger. This maneuver can also be applied to the deep muscles such as the musculaus rectus of the back. Sometimes it is done by lifting and letting go of the muscle with the tip of the thumb and index finger.

Main points observed: When the deep muscle of the back (above and below Gaohuang, B 43) is lifted, the forearm of the patient must be turned to the lower back to make the back relax. Otherwise the muscle cannot be gripped.

Functions: It is used to activate *qi* and blood circulation on the back, alleviate contracture and dispel pathogenic cold and wind.

19. Percussing Maneuver (See Fig. 2-30)

This is done by the doctor with a finger-bent palm, a loose fist, a lateral palm, the back of the hand or the two palms put together. The back and limbs are usually percussed by a curved palm or a loose fist, and the head and abdomen are often percussed by a lateral palm, the back of the hand and the palms put together.

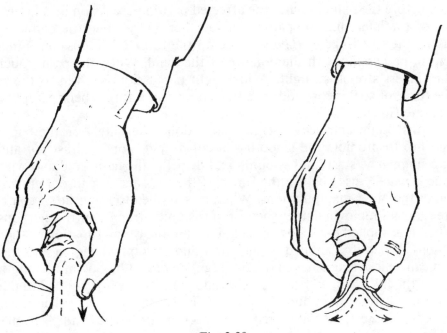

Fig. 2-29

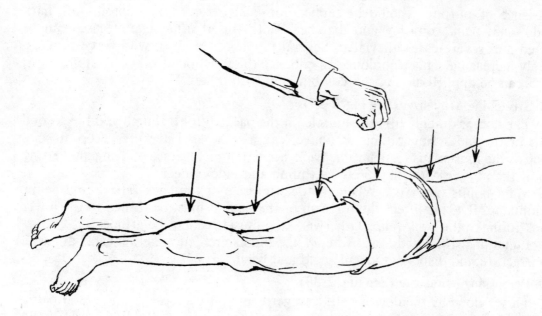

Fig. 2-30

Main points observed: Percussion is done forcefully. The five fingers are separated before the palm touches the affected part in percussion by a lateral palm, the back of the hand and the palms put together. Only when the palm percusses the muscle, the five fingers come to close on the force of percussion. Fingers are first bent in percussion with the dorsum of the hand. When the palm touches the skin, the fingers stretch straight. A just right percussion is given to the muscles since the force of striking is moderate by a loose fist, a finger-bent palm or a palm with separate fingers.

Functions: Light and heavy percussion is done alternately on the back, lower back and hip to promote the smooth flow of *qi* and blood, adjust *yin* and *yang*, eliminate stagnancy, stasis and swelling and dispel pathogenic cold and wind. This technique is usually used before the finish of the massage, because it enhances the function of the other manipulations. When it is applied to the head, it can refresh, alleviate pain by removing stagnancy or stasis, and strengthen the nervous function. When it is applied to the lower back, it can improve the function of the kidney and tendons. When it is applied to the chest and abdominal region and the costal region, it can relieve stagnancy and pain, regulate *qi* and blood, and strengthen the function of the liver, help *qi* flow and alleviate pain. When it is applied to the chest, it can alleviate cardiac pain due to spasm of the cardiac vessels. When the chest is percussed, the loose fist should strike the back of the hand which is put on the chest. Three to five percussions are enough to dredge the heart Meridian and

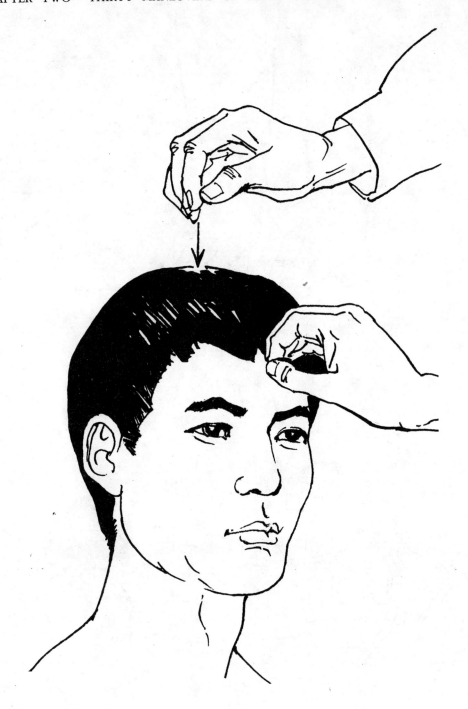

Fig. 2-31

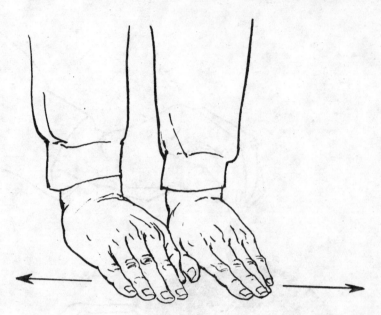

Fig. 2-32a

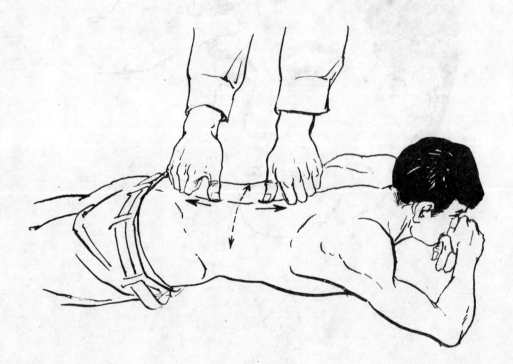

Fig. 2-32b

alleviate a suffocating feeling.

20. Puncturing Maneuver (See Fig. 2-31)

It is done by the doctor to stimulate the scalp, frontal, eye orbit, and zygomatic bone.

Main points observed: The finger nails must be regularly cut and not too sharp so as not to hurt the skin. On puncturing the frontal and eyebrow region, the manipulation starts from Yintang (Extra 1) or Zanzhu (B 2) to the lateral part; on puncturing of the scalp, the manipulation starts from the posterior to anterior or vice versa. Light and forceful puncture is applied alternately.

Functions: It is used to refresh oneself, remove dizziness and is usually applied to superficial muscles.

21. Separating Maneuver (See Fig. 2-32)

The doctor pushes in a contrary direction by the pad of the thumbs or middle fingers, usually applied to the umbilicus region, lower back and forhead, when pushing the forehead the two fingers move from the eyebrow bone to both temples.

Functions: This technique is used to eliminate stagnancy and stasis, stimulate blood circulation and help muscles and tendons to relax, regulate *qi* and blood and relieve spasms and pain. This technique is usually used in injuries of the lumbar muscles, together with the pressing maneuver, and in spastic intussusception. The technique is also used to alleviate headaches and hernia.

22. Joining Maneuver (See Fig. 2-33)

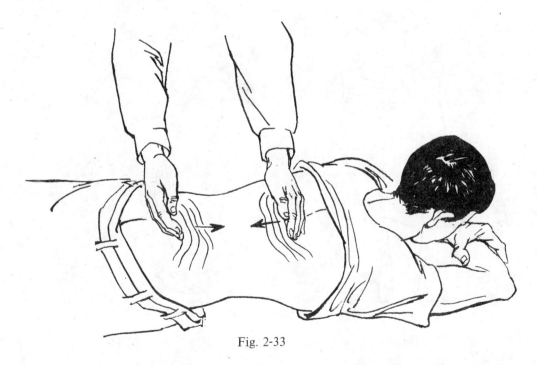

Fig. 2-33

The doctor drives his two hands close, usually applied to the umbilicus region, in an up and down or right and left movement. This technique is usually used together with the two-hand pushing maneuver. The former is the reinforcing method and the latter the reducing method. In general, the joining maneuver is applied first, then the two-hand pushing maneuver, i.e., more reinforcing and less reducing.

Functions: It is used to reinforce the spleen and stomach and replenish *qi*, promote digestion and warm up the umbilicus region. The umbilicus tends to be affected by pathogenic wind and as a result diseases occur owing to pathogenic factors. This manipulation is applied to expel pathogenic wind, and reinforce the spleen, stomach and kidney. Digestion is activated because the small intestine is located in the umbilicus region. Therefore it is important to use the method in treatment of abdominal conditions.

23. Back-carrying Maneuver (See Figs. 2-34/35)

The doctor stands back to back with the patient and lifts him on to his back.

Main points observed: The doctor must hold the patient tightly when he tries to carry the patient on his back. His feet must be separated in line with his shoulders. When the patient is being carried on the back of the doctor, the crown

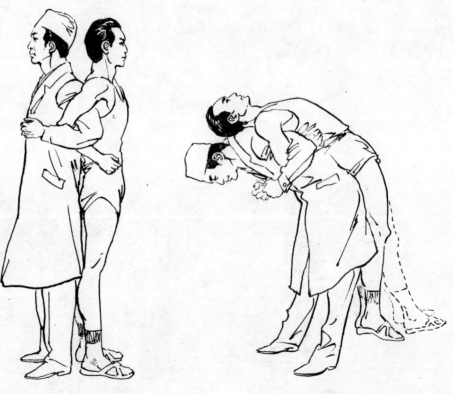

Fig. 2-34   Fig. 2-35

of his head should be close to the doctor's nape and his feet are loosely hanging. At this moment the doctor moves his hip a few times and moves right and left to strengthen the action of traction. It is usually used to treat prolapse of the lumbar intervertebral disc and other lumbar injuries. My clinical experience has shown that this method is effective in treatment of lumbar conditions and leg pain. The advantages are as follows: (1) safe—I often use this method to treat lumbago with unknown causes and those cases of prolapse of the lumbar intervertabral disc to which traction cannot be applied. The traction is done by the patient's own weight and there are no side-effects. In the beginning the doctor bends slightly for a short time. When there is no pain he may bend more for long time; (2) simple; (3) effective— In some cases, lumbago is difficult to cure. There is contracture of the greater psoas muscle, anterior longitudinal ligament and posterior longitudinal ligament. Only this method is useful because muscles behind the abdominal cavity and in front of the vertebrae cannot be touched by other manipulations.

24. Holding Maneuver (See Figs. 2-36/37)

The doctor holds the patient in his arms from behind with the patient's hands on his and lifts him so that the patient's feet naturally touch the ground.

Main points observed: In doing it, the doctor's feet should be apart, and when the patient is lifted, his feet just loosely touch the ground. The patient should also be jolted and shaken a bit.

Functions: This technique is a kind of traction using the patient's own weight, usually applied to cases of pain in the lower back and thigh. But this method is

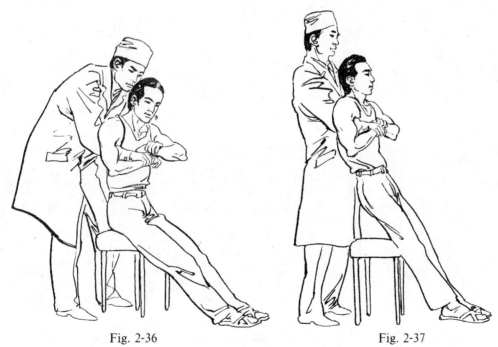

Fig. 2-36   Fig. 2-37

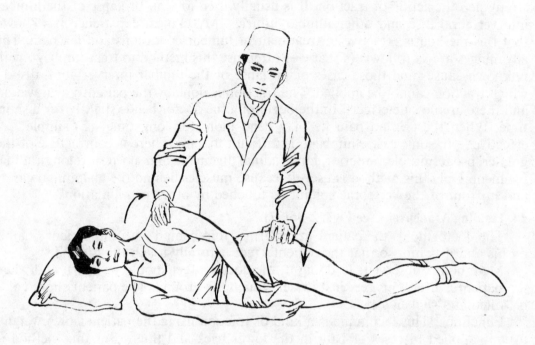

Fig. 2-38

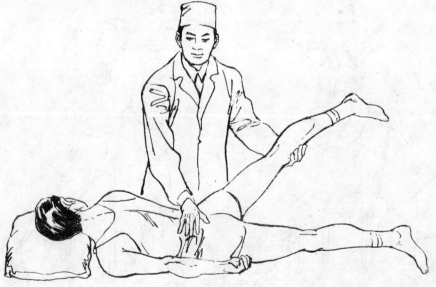

Fig. 2-39

not frequently used.

25. Pulling Maneuver (See Figs. 2-38/39)

The doctor presses a part of the patient's body with one hand and pulls another part with the other hand to rotate or stretch a dislocated or transpositive joint. It is usually applied to the lower back, limbs and neck.

Main points observed: The patient is in a lateral recumbent position with the affected part upward. The doctor stands behind him and presses the back of his shoulder with one hand, and the anterior superior iliac spine with the other, then he turns the shoulder forward and makes the anterior superior iliac spine move backward. When he is exerting his top strength, the doctor suddenly turns the patient's lower back forcefully and a cracking sound is heard. The manipulation is completed.

Functions: It is used to stimulate the circulation of blood and relax the muscle, and remove adhesion and dislocation to restore the function of the joint.

26. Kneading Maneuver (See Figs. 2-40/41)

The doctor pokes the inferior or medial contracture or oilsthy muscle tendon, or the adhesive muscle tendons with his thumb with the help of his other hand. Sometimes a fist is put in the patient's armpit to open the adhesion and the manipulation is done.

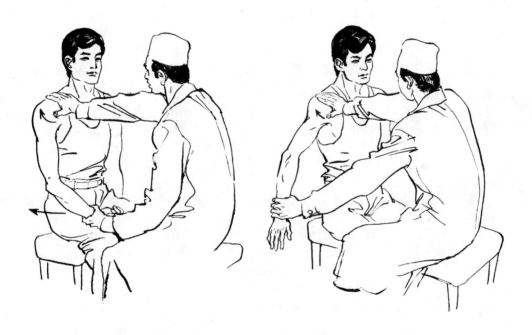

Fig. 2-40   Fig. 2-41

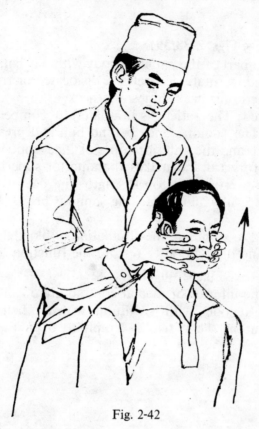

Fig. 2-42

Functions: It is used to alleviate spasm and pain, and soft adhesive tissue.

27. Head-lifting Maneuver (See Fig. 2-42)

The doctor lifts the head of the patient a little with both hands. This technique is different from the bone-reduction maneuver. The doctor presses the part above Fenchi (B 20) with the pads of his thumb and with the middle finger situated below Taiyang (Extra 2) and the heart of the palm on the ear. Then the patient's head is gradually lifted.

Functions: This method is used to pull the cervical vertebrae and to treat cervical disorders and stiff neck.

Main points observed: After the completion of other manipulations, this method is applied. The doctor should stand close behind the patient and lift his head straight upward with moderate force. Only the muscle of the neck is pulled, the patient's body should not be lifted.

28. Raising Maneuver (See Figs. 2-43/44)

This is an adjunct manipulation rather than an independent maneuver. For example, when other manipulations are applied to the shoulder of the patient, the doctor asks him to put his arm on his shoulder and raise it as much as possible.

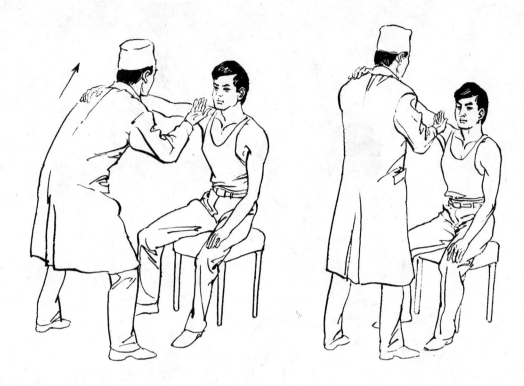

Fig. 2-43   Fig. 2-44

Main points observed: The doctor should stand facing the patient, who is sitting on a chair. The patient stretches his arm and puts his hand on the doctor's shoulder. When he is pressing and rolling on the patient's muscles of the anterior shoulder and armpit in bent position, the doctor gradually straightens his back to raise the patient's arm up.

Functions: This technique is used to alleviate the adhesive joint, and restore its function. It is painless and better than a forceful traction.

29. Lifting Maneuver (See Fig. 2-45)

The doctor lifts the patient's arm, the muscle lift has already been discussed above. Here the stress is only on lifting the arm. The patient is in a sitting position with his affected arm in front of the chest. The fingers are held upward with the palm facing the chest. The doctor stands in front of the patient and holds the patient's five fingers with both hands. He makes clockwise and counterclockwise movements to turn the shoulder joint. Then he lifts the patient's arm suddenly and forcefully.

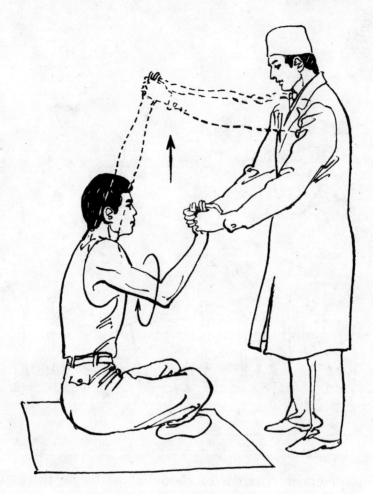

Fig. 2-45

Functions: It is used to activate the smooth flow of *qi* and blood, stimulate blood circulation and help the muscles and tendons to relax in order to improve the joint function of the arm and shoulder.

30. Stepping Maneuver (See Fig. 2-46)

The doctor steps on the affected part of the patient with one foot or both feet and moves his heel up and down. Kneading and pushing is given by the foot at the same time. It is usually applied to the lower back and sacrum to treat prolapse of lumbar intervertebral disc with strong pressure.

Main points observed: For a strong and big figured patient the method is often used when the doctor's force is not enough to exert its effect. First the doctor should experiment on healthy people to gain experience in the technique, and then apply it clinically. It is seldom used for other parts of the body.

Functions: It is used to activate the smooth flow of *qi* and blood, helping the muscles and tendons to relax.

The above are thirty commonly-used manipulations. When a doctor knows them, it is not difficult to learn other maneuvers.

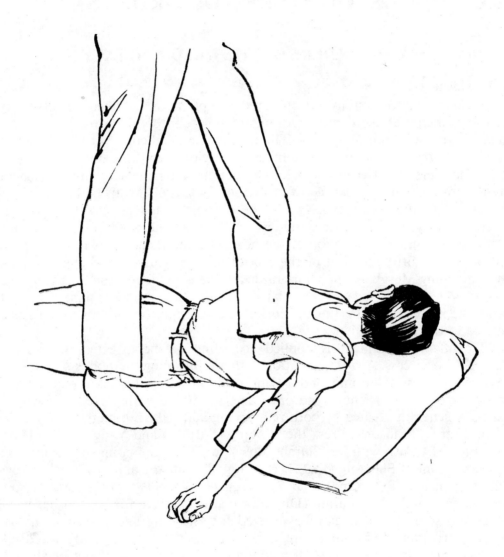

Fig. 2-46

CHAPTER THREE
TUINA TREATMENT OF COMMONLY ENCOUNTERED DISORDERS

I. DISORDERS OF THE HEAD AND FACE

1. Headache

Headache, a commonly encountered symptom, is ascribed to a variety of factors, which are regarded in traditional Chinese medicine as exogeneous pathogenic factors and internal injury. The former are wind-cold, wind-heat and wind-dampness, while the latter include hyperactivity of liver yang, phlegm-turbidity, *qi* deficiency, blood deficiency and kidney deficiency. In general, the headache of short duration is mostly caused by affection of the exogeneous pathogenic factors, pertaining to the excess type, while the chronic headache mostly results from internal injury, pertaining to deficiency. Clinically, the differentiation should be made according to the location of the headache and its accompanying symptoms. According to differentiation of the meridians, the frontal headache is related to the Yangming Meridian; the temporal headache is related to the Shaoyang Meridian; the occipital headache is related to the Taiyang Meridian; the vertical headache is related to the Jueyin Meridian; and headache radiating to the back is related to the Du Meridian.

Treatment: Treatment is applied according to the affected meridians and deficiency or excess. A sitting position with a reinforcing method is selected in the case of an excess syndrome, and a lying position with a reducing method is used in the case of a dificiency syndrome. The syndrome with mixed dificiency and excess is generally treated by both reinforcing and reducing methods.

1) Frontal headache: Press the Yintang (Extra 1) and Yangbai (G 14) points (See Fig. 3-1). Push with the thumbs alternately from the point of Yintang (Extra 1) to the point of Shenting (Du 24) (See Fig. 3-2) at the anterior hairline for two minutes. In addition, Zanzhu (B 2), Hegu (LI 4), bilateral Taiyang (Extra 2), Shangxing (Du 23) and Baihui (Du 20) are also effective for frontal headache. If necessary, some of them may, be selected for kneading and pressing. In case of nasal obstruction and running nose, digital pressing of the Yingxiang (LI 20) point is added (See Fig. 3-3). In case of a cough due to cold phlegm, the Feishu (B 13) and Lieque (L 7) points are pushed, pressed, kneaded and rubbed with the fingers and palms.

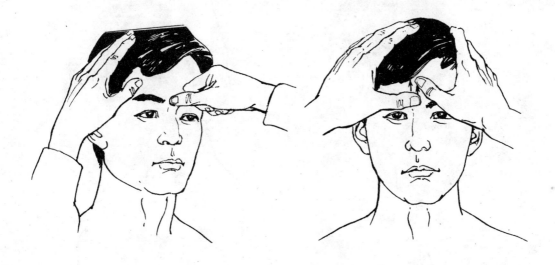

Fig. 3-1   Fig. 3-2

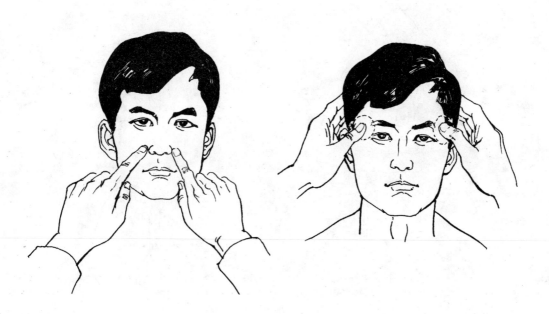

Fig. 3-3   Fig. 3-4

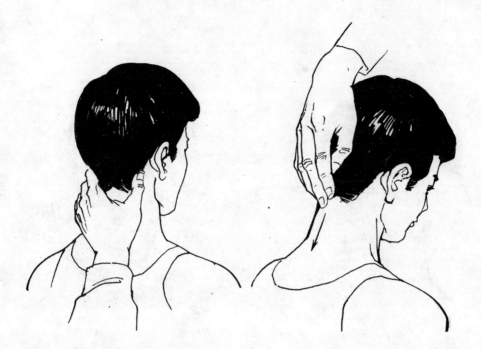

Fig. 3-5   Fig. 3-6

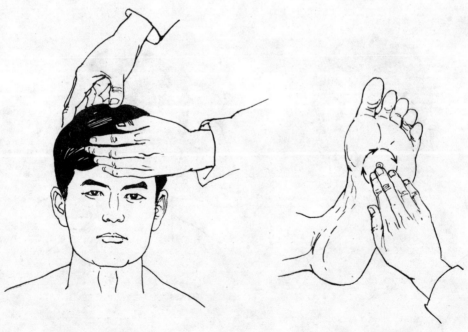

Fig. 3-7   Fig. 3-8

2) Temporal headache: Principally press and palm-rub the Taiyang (Extra 2) point (See Fig. 3-4), grasp and push the Fengchi (B 20) point on both sides of the nape and its upper and lower portions. The Fengchi (B 20), point may be excessively kneaded (See Fig. 3-5) and pressed to improve the shortage of blood supply to the head until slight sweating appears, which may not only eliminate the wind, but also resolve the dampness, however only profuse sweating is able to eliminate the wind. In addition, the points Touwei (S 8), Tongziliao (G 1), Sizhukong (SJ 23) and Yanglingquan (G 34) are also effective for temporal headache. If necessary, pressing and kneading of these points may be added. Push and pinch the midline from Fengfu (Du 16) to Dazhui (Du 14) at the posterior nape with more pushings. (See Fig. 3-6). The upward pushing is reinforcing, while the downward pushing is reducing.

3) Occipital headache: Principally push and press the Fengchi (G 20) and Fengfu (Du 16) points, in combination with the Touwei (S 8), Shangxing (Du 23), Shuaigu (G 8) and Hegu (LI 4) points.

4) Vertical headache: Principally press the Baihui (Du 20) and Yongquan (K 1) points (See Figs. 3-7/8) with the thumb. Pressing Baihui (Du 20) helps *qi* ascend, relieves pain and clears the mind in case of headache and dizziness due to hypotension, while pressing Yongquan (K 1) may help *qi* descend and alleviate pain. The points of Dicang (S 4), Hegu (LI 4), Renzhong (Du 26), Touwei (S 8) and Jiache (S 6) may be selected symptomatically.

5) Headache radiating to the back: Principally press and push the Dazhui (Du 14) point inferior to the nape, in combination with packing-up of both to Zanzhu (B 2) point (See Fig. 3-9) and pushing the Yintang (Extra) point. Grasp the Jianjing (G 21) point, roll the two large tendons on the back, press and knead the tender points and slightly stroke the back.

6) Headache due to hypertension: Headache accompanied by dizziness and

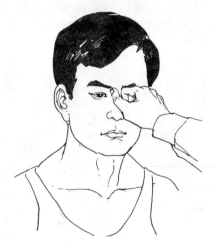

Fig. 3-9

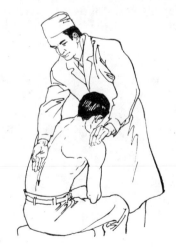

Fig. 3-10

distending pain is mostly the excess syndrome, which is principally treated by palm-rubbing the bilateral Taiyang (Extra) point with the reducing method, followed by pushing along the Du Meridian from the points of Dazhui (Du 14) to Changqiang (Du 1) with the lateral palm (See Fig. 3-10). Press and knead Yongquan (K 1) and grasp Kunlun (B 60). (See Fig. 3-11). If necessary, pressing Yintang (Extra 2), Touwei (S 8), Lieque (L 7) and Hegu (LI 4) may be combined. Grasp Fengchi (G 20) with the reducing method.

7) Neurasthenic headache: Headache is only limited in the forehead, vertex and temporal region with mild pain and some dizziness. It mostly pertains to the deficiency type, which may be treated according to the routine method for headache with the reinforcing method, i.e., push, press, knead and grasp Yintang (Extra 1), Taiyang (Extra 2), Yangbai (G 14), Fengchi (G 20) and Hegu (LI 4) respectively, then pick up Zanzhu (B 2) with the thumb and index fingertips, wipe along the superciliary arch from Yintang (Extra 1) to Zanzhu (B 2), Yuyao (Extra 3), and Sizhukong (SJ 23), then puncture the forehead with the fingertips, percuss the head with the lateral palm first and then with the back of the finger. Between manipulations, comb the scalp with the ten fingers (See Fig. 3-12), which may refresh the mind, brighten the eyesight, clear the head and relieve pain.

8) Trigeminal neuralgia: Severe pain like cutting, burning and electric shock in paraxysmal attacks, occurring mostly at the temple region, results from wind, fire, phlegm or stagnation, pertaining to the excess type. The effect when treated by *tuina* therapy is not so fast as that with acupuncture, but pain can be relieved. Increasing treatments can also strengthen the effect. In general, heavy pressing, pushing and grasping of the points of Hegu (LI 4), Jiache (S 6), Xiaguan (S 7), Dicang (S 4), Neiting (S 44), Zulinqi (G 4), and pressing Ashi is effective.

Typical Case: A woman aged 34 suffered from headache for more than ten years and medication failed to resolve the problem. The pain was intermittent and not so severe and not at a fixed location. An EEG showed normal results. She came to the clinic on July 18, 1983 and neurathenic headache was diagnosed. The pain

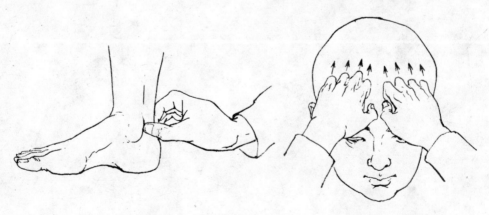

Fig. 3-11   Fig. 3-12

was relieved by applying the manipulation 1) or 2) for treatment, but she still had frequent attacks of headache. *Tuina* treatment was performed when the headache came. After many continuous treatment she was completely cured.

2. Toothache

Toothache is a commonly encountered symptom, and is divided into fire toothache, dental caries, unstable dental alveolus and pain due to a loose tooth according to its etiology. In general, pressing the point Hegu (LI 4) with the fingernail may check pain (See Fig. 3-13). In case of severe pain, pressing and kneading the points of Quanliao (SI 18), Xiaguan (S 7) and Shaohai (H 3) (See Fig. 3-14), may be added. In case of persistent pain, pressing the points Taiyang (Extra 2) and Jiache (S 6) is added. Press the left side in case of pain in the left side and vice versa. (See Fig. 3-15). If necessary, it is advisable to press Ermen (SJ 21) (upper toothache), Shangyang (LI 1), Erjian (LI 2), Sanjian (LI 3) (lower toothache), Yangxi (LI 5) and Taixi (K 3).

Loose tooth, dental cavity, toothache occurring during eating are due to the stimulation of the root nerves which is treated by extracting the dead tooth. In this way toothache may be temporarily relieved; but the teeth close to the extracted tooth may be loosened, and toothache will occur again. Then the diseased tooth has to be extracted, therefore, it is not appropriate to this mothod. Extraction of one tooth will lead to the loosening of another one. However, pressing Quanliao (SI 18), Xiaguan(S 7), Jiache (S 6) and Hegu (LI 4) to treat toothache is a good method. The best way is to have an early denture making to prevent tooth loosening of the extraction.

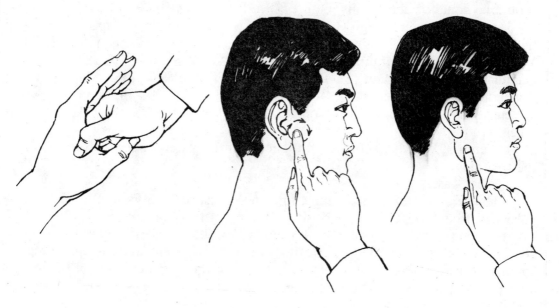

Fig. 3-13   Fig. 3-14   Fig. 3-15

3. Facial Paralysis

Facial paralysis, also known as deviation of the mouth and eyes and facial nerve palsy, is a commonly encountered disease, appearing mostly in the elderly, and sometimes in the middle-aged and children. Chinese medecine ascribes this condition to wind-cold attacking the meridians. The onset is abrupt and one-sided numbness and paralysis, inability to frown, raise the forehead, expose the teeth and blow, deviation of the mouth corner to the healthy side, failure in closing the eyelids, shallowing of the nasolabial sulcus, and disappearance of partial wrinkles may be found in the morning after waking up. If *tuina* treatment is given in time, better results will be achieved. Those with a longer history of the disease will have lesser effects, but some symptoms can be relieved. The treatment is directed to dispel wind, clear and activate the meridians, promote blood circulation to remove blood stasis, and warm the skin to eliminate cold.

Treatment:

1) The patient is asked to sit down and the doctor stands behind the patient facing his back. He must wash his hands before starting the manipulation. When the hands are still wet after cleaning, the doctor stretches out both his hands from the patient's back to rub and knead the patient's face from below to above in order to strengthen the elasity of the face muscle and minimize the wrinkles for about two minutes. (See Fig. 3-16).

2) Apply slight picking-up, kneading and rubbing manipulations on the face with emphasis on the affected side. In case of small painful nodules around the points Xiaguan (S 7) and Jiache (S 6) on the affected side, kneading and picking-up should be done for about four minutes (See Figs. 3-17/19).

3) Grasp the points Hegu (LI 4), Fengchi (G 20), and Jianjing (G 21), pick-up the points Zanzhu (B 2), bilaterally , digitally and press the points Yifeng (SJ 17), Yintang (Extra 1), Jingming (B 1), Tongziliao (G 1) (See Fig. 3-20), Sibai (S 2), Quanliao (SI 18), Xiaguan (S 7), Jiache (S 6), Dicang (S 4), Yingxiang (LI 20), Renzhong (Du 26), Chengjiang (Ren 24) and Baihui (Du 20). Press mostly on the affected side. Digital pressing is sometimes applied on the healthy side for about seven minutes.

4) Percuss the head, shoulder and back with the lateral palm before finishing the treatment.

Typical Case:

A teacher, aged 37 came to the clinic on August 5, 1975 with left facial nerve palsy due to an attack by wind during sleeping in the countryside in 1964. After the treatment, some improvements were obtained, but a relapse occurred on June 20, 1981. She was admitted to the hospital for treatment and the pathological conditions were relieved, but incomplete closing of the eyes, deviation of the mouth and a daily paraxysmal numb feeling on the affected side remained. The first treatment was given on August 5 according to the above-mentioned method, in which gentle, rapid and soft manipulations were carried out to excite the nerves

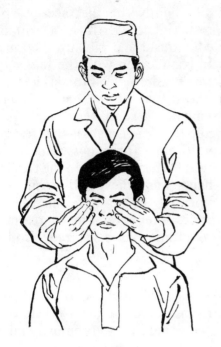

Fig. 3-16

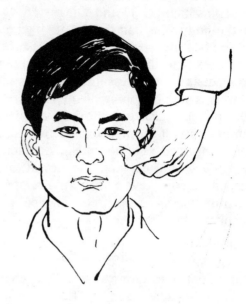

Fig. 3-17

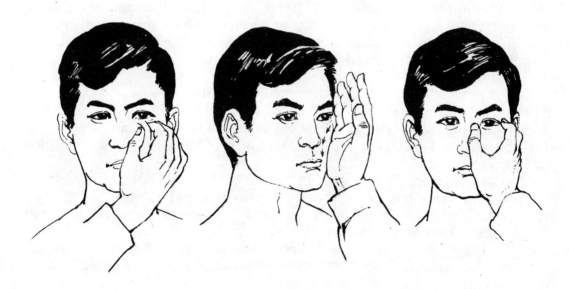

Fig. 3-18   Fig. 3-19   Fig. 3-20

and promote the blood circulation. First of all, slightly rub the face, grasp the points Fengchi (G 20) and Jianjing (G 21), press Yintang (Extra 1), Jingming (B 1), Tongziliao (G 1) and Dicang (S 4) repeatedly knead and pick-up the museles at the point Xiaguan (S 7) and Jiache (S 6). In comparison with the face muscle on the healthy side, spasm, nodules and severe pain were felt on the affected side. Repeated kneading and slight rubbing with the thenar of the hand should be applied, and then pressing the points of Yingxiang (LI 20) and Renzhong (Du 26), as well as slight rubbing of the face are followed before the finish of the treatment. The patient said that she had not felt so comfortable for many years and the temperature of the affected side was also improved. Afterwards when the treatment was continued several times, the facial numbness was relieved, the complexion restored to normal and the deviation was improved. Because the massage was suspended for a few days, a mild relapse took place. After several more treatments, the numbness disappeared. The patient recovered and has discharged from the hospital.

4. Insomnia

Insomnia is manifested by difficulty in falling asleep, inablity to sleep, abnormal wakefulness, or disturbed sleep with dreams accompanied by listlessness, dizziness, headache, indigestion, poor appetite, hypomnesia, and seminal emission and impotence in males. This condition results from insufficiency of the heart and spleen, disharmony between the heart and kidney, *qi* deficiency of the heart and gallbladder, or disturbance of the descending function of the stomach due to phlegm-fire or food retention. Western medicine ascribes this condition to a functional disturbance of the nervous system. The methods of treatment are many, such as Western medications and Chinese herbs, acupuncture and moxibustion. *Tuina* is effective in treating insomnia, especially good for those who have used medication even a longer period of time without success.

Treatment:

In light of the above-mentioned method for treating headache, some appropriate manipulations are added or reduced to treat headache and dizziness. A chiropractic treatment is performed on the patient's lower back and back.

1) Slightly stroke the back with the palms of both hands from above to below three times.

2) Grasp the point Jianjing (G 21) bilaterally (See Fig. 3-21), then press the Shu points corresponding to the Zang-Fu organs and the important points along the Bladder Meridian on both sides from above to below. After pressing, slightly stroke three times. (See Fig. 3-22)

3) First grasp the Jianjing (G 21) point and then press and stroke the Shu points and the important points of the Bladder Meridian bilaterally with the thenar of the palm from above to below three times each.

4) Press Shenshu (B 23), Qihaishu (B 24), Dachangshu (B 25), Guanyuanshu (B 26), Baihuanshu (B 30), Shangliao (B 31), Ciliao (B 32), Zhongliao (B 33),

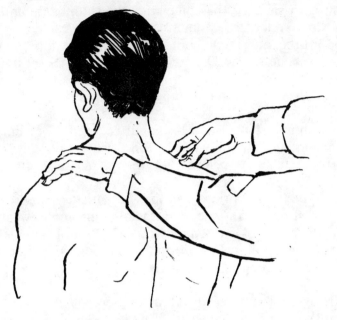

Fig. 3-21

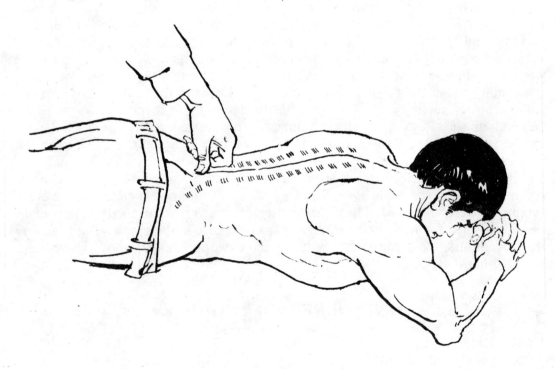

Fig. 3-22

Xialiao (B 34) on both sides of the spine with the thumbs of both hands. After pressing, slightly stroke once, three times, three minutes each. (See Fig. 3-23).

5) Pick up and lift the muscles on both sides of the spine along the Du Meridian from the coccysacral bone to the Dazhui (Du 14) point. (See Fig. 3-24). Slightly stroke with the palm of the thumb from the points of Dazhui (Du 14) to Changqiang (Du 1) several *cun* lateral to the spine three times before finishing the treatment.

6) Percuss the scapula, spine, lower back, buttock and lower limbs respectively with the fist, palm and lateral palm with the force using a lighter, force each time. Slightly stroke from above to below with the palms of both hands crossing alternately.

Insomnia should be treated prior to sleep. The patient is advised not to smoke or drink tea prior to sleeping. In case of intractable insomnia, wash the feet with hot water and do not read books which may cause nervous excitement. After *tuina* manipulations, the patient will feel comfortable and soon fall asleep. Some patients fall asleep during the treatment and sleep very soundly.

Typical Case:

A female cadre aged 51 came to the clinic on September 12, 1983. The patient had a sallow complexion and was emaciated with sluggish eyes, a low voice and chronic pain. Chief complaints: insomnia, dizziness, headache, depression of the chest, intercostal pain, muscle and joint pain, irritability, hot temper, preference for quietness, loss of appetite, slight red urine, normal stools, string-taut, thready and rapid pulse, yellow coating, red borders of the tongue, abnormal menstruation before menopause, one hour sleep at night, excessive dreaming and lassitude. She was treated in several hospitals without any effects. Especially in the last two years, the condition had been aggravated because her husband died. Diognosis: depression (neurosis, disturbance of the vegetative nerves) and menopausal syndrome. General massage was applied according to the above-mentioned method with emphasis on the chest, back and head. After the first treatment, she felt comfortable, clear-minded and her eyes brightened. After the third treatment, the dizziness and headache were relieved, her sleep increased, and her appetite improved. After seven treatments, she could sleep for more than four hours, eat rice, and the other symptoms were alleviated. The massage treatments were continued another eight times, and then the headache and dizziness disappeared. She could sleep for more than five hours, the dreams were reduced and her appetite was good. The patient resumed her daily work.

II. DISORDERS OF THE NECK

1. Stiffneck

Stiffneck results from long hyperextension of the cervical muscle due to an improper sleep position, leading to a protective reflex spasm. This case may also

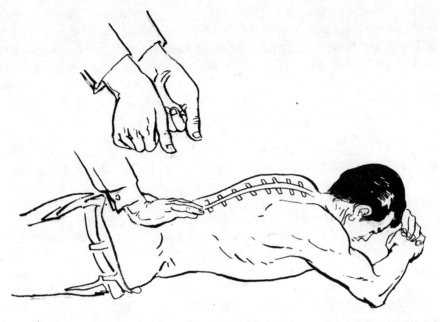

Fig. 3-23

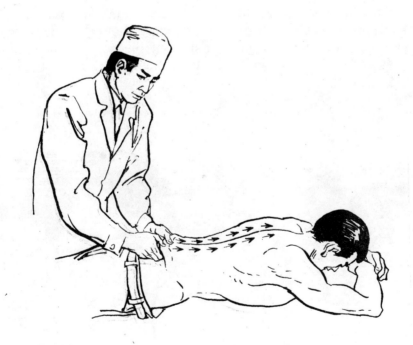

Fig. 3-24

be caused by wind-cold attacking the neck, or by trauma. The symptoms are soreness and pain in the neck, difficulty in shaking the head. The pain rediates to the affected shoulder, back and upper limbs, In severe cases, the head tilts to either side, and tenderness appears on the affected side of the neck. A mild case may gradually recover without treatment, but can be quickly cured with immediate treatment, while severe cases should be treated in time, and immediate effects can be achieved.

Treatment:

The patient is in a sitting position and the doctor stands behind him, showing his hand posterior-laterally to lead the patient's head to move upon the movement of the hand in order to move the patient's neck. Anteflexion and retroversion of 35° is normal and for the left and right rotation 45° is normal. The limitation and appearance of pain are considered as disease (See Figs. 3-25/26). Pressing, kneading, pushing, rolling, grasping and rubbing maneuvers at the neck, nape and back muscles may assure safe, painless and quick treatment.

1) The patient should be in a sitting position and the doctor stands behind him. Slightly stroke from the nape to the bilateral shoulders and back with both hands several times to relax the neck and nape muscles.

2) Grasp and knead the Jianjing (G 21) point with one hand or both hands with the force gradually increasing to eliminate or reduce the contracture of the nuchal muscles for two to three minutes until the muscles of the shoulder and nape are relaxed or comparatively relaxed. The thick muscle of the spina scapulae should not be wrongly diagnosed as contracture, and kneading should not be done there.

3) Grasp and knead the muscles on both sides of the neck from the Fengchi (G 20) point to the root of the nape with the alternating hand. Supporting the head

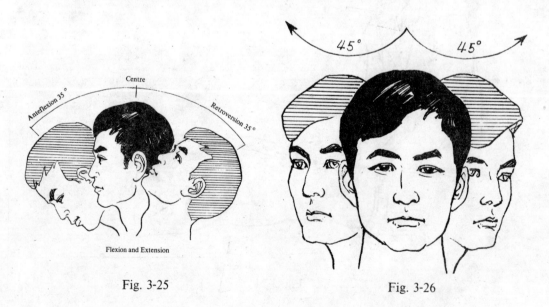

Fig. 3-25   Fig. 3-26

with four fingers, press and poke the Yifeng (SJ 17) point with the thumb. (See Fig. 3-27)

4) Press and knead the Jianwaishu (SI 14) (See Fig. 3-28), Tianzong (SI 11), Bingfeng (SI 12) points and the nearby tender points with the thumb.

5) Ask the patient to tilt his face upward slightly to relax the nuchal muscles. Pick up the nuchal muscle from the Dazhui (Du 14) point to the Fengfu (Du 16) point. In case of tightness of the nuchal muscle, pushing of the nape from above to below is applied several times instead (The doctor should stand in front of the patient, and the patient should bow his head).

6) Before finishing the treatment, tap and percuss the shoulders and scapulae, and then slightly stroke them several times. In this way, the muscles of the neck, nape, sternoclavicle and scapula are relaxed and stiffneck is relieved. Some remaining symptoms can be naturally relieved.

Typical Case:

A male worker aged 32 came to the clinic on August 17, 1973, and complained of stiffneck, associated with pain aggravated on exertion, limitation of rotation and upward bending of the head, and inability to walk. He did not pay attention to the case because he thought he would recover naturally. Five days had passed before the condition was aggravated. Then he came to see the doctor. Examination: Unbearable pain upon touching the neck. The above-mentioned method was applied and stiffneck was cured very soon.

2. Cervical Spondylopathy

Cervical spondylopathy, also known as cervical syndrome, is a commonly encountered disease of the middle-aged and elderly. This disease mostly results from the retrograde affection of the cervical intervertebral disc and the surrounding soft tissues, such as degeneration of the cervical intervertebral disc, elastic reduction or outward protrusion of the cervical intervertebral disc, narrowing of intervertebral space, hyperosteogeny of the pyramidal border, malposition of the intervertebral facet joint, reduction of the vertebral foramen, disappearance of physiological bent; degeneration, thickening, hardening, calcification and ossification of yellow ligament and the nuchal ligament. Some cases are due to trauma or overstrain (physical labour at the hyperextension position for too long), leading to malposition of the cervical vertebral facet joint, injury of soft tissues, such as bleeding, swelling, and adhesion. In mild cases, there may be pain, numbness of the head, neck, nape, shoulder and the arm and musculor atrophy, while in severe cases, there may be intense pain, inability to rotate and bend upward, and even hemiplegia.

Treatment:

This case may be basically cured or greatly improved after *tuina* treatment. Prior to treatment, the details of etiology, case history, course of disease and symptoms should be well understood. In addition to the examination for stiffneck mentioned above, the other examinations such as brachial plexus catatasis, pressure

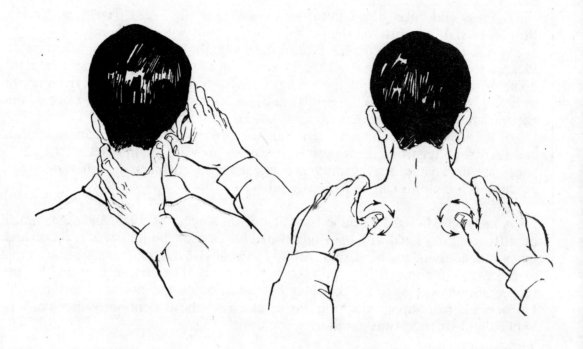

Fig. 3-27   Fig. 3-28

test of the vertebral foramen (See Figs. 3-29/30), gripping strength test and x-ray test should be added. The patient should be in a sitting position and the doctor stands behind the patient.

1) Comb the scalp with the 10 fingers, slightly stroke the muscles and skin of the neck, nape, shoulders and back, grasp and knead the shoulder tendons to relax the muscles.

2) Grasp and knead the neck muscle with both hands alternately with the same manipulation as that for stiffneck.

3) Knead both sides of the neck with the thumbs of both hands respectively from above to below for a few minutes. The finger force should be gradually increased. Then roll and knead the muscle of the nape and shoulder either with the thenar of the hand or with the forearm. Knead for a few minutes (A large and thick tendon cramp or muscle may be touched under the fingers in case of severe contracture, which is different from the healthy side. The kneading time should be longer.)

4) Press and knead the Yifeng (SJ 17), Jianwaishu (SI 14), Tianzong (SI 11), Bingfeng (SI 12), Tianrong (SI 17), and Jianjing (G 21) points with the palm and the thenar of the fingers, with emphasis on some obvious tender

points. Knead and press Jianwaishu (SI 14) with the thumb for a longer time and good results will be achieved, which are similar to those for bone setting. Therefore, the dislocation and malposition of the vertebra are related to the degenerative contracture and the muscle tension. If only the dislocation is corrected, but the normal functions of the muscles are not restored, the bone setting effect is not stable because dislocation may occur again due to muscle tension. Treatment is directed to relax the muscular spasm and promote the circulation of qi and blood, which helps stabilize the bone setting effects. Press and knead the muscular contracture at the media-superior angle of the scapula and double effects will be achieved. For semiluxation of the cervical vertebra with a history of fracture, the manipulation is very difficult. For the sake of safety, knead the Shu-points of the shoulder a lot instead of bone setting. With this method the results should be satisfactory, pain should disappear, and the functions greatly improve.

5) Lift the nape and the neck two to three times.

6) Grasp the subaxillary posterior and anterior muscle groups (i.e., the middle finger touching the Zhongji Ren 3 point, the thumb pressing the Jianzhen, SI 9 point), press the Jianyu (SI 15) and Binao (LI 14) points, grasp the Quchi (LI 11), Shousanli (LI 10) and Hegu (LI 4) points, grasp the medial and lateral muscles of the upper limbs from the wrist to the armpit, twist, grip and flick the finger joints.

7) Slightly tap, percuss and stroke all the areas being treated.

8) The same or a simple manipulation may be applied to the healthy arm.

Typical Case:

A male cadre aged 52 came to the clinic in the spring of 1977, and complained of problems with the cervical vertebra for three years. Hyperosteogeny, and narrowing of the vertebra space were found at the cervical vertebrae Nos. four, five and six in the x-ray examination. The condition was worsening, accompanied by stiffneck, severe pain, inability to rotate the head, numbness of the fingers on one side, and insomnia. Disease of the cervical vertebra was diagnosed in one hospital, and treated according to the above-mentioned manipulations. After being treated by the trial light manipulation for 15 minutes, the neck was able to rotate, but poorly on the left side. The next day the patient said he had slept soundly for about five hours at night. The pain was greatly relieved, but the fingers still remained numb. Then the treatment continued two times according to the above-mentioned method, but the finger force was a little increased. After that, the neck function was basically recovered, he could sleep soundly for six hours, his appetite increased, and the pain disappeared. Only some soreness remained. Numbness of the fingers was also relieved. In order to strengthen the effect, the patient was taught to do some exercises. The follow-up visit three years later found no relapse and he was able to resume his work.

III. PERIARTHRITIS OF THE SHOULDER

Periarthritis of the shoulder, a frequently encountered disease, is related to a weak constitution due to old age, insufficient of *qi* and blood, and not enough nourishment of the tendons and vessels. This disease often occurs around the age of 50. In addition, this condition is also closely related to carrying heavy loads, frequent movement, hyperactivity or hypoactivity of the shoulder joint, heavy lifting or sudden rotation, and direct impact with external objects. After injury, there may be local blood stasis, swelling, pain and motor limitation. In case of delayed treatment, tissue adhesion may result. Under such conditions heavy labour will worsen the adhesion of the shoulder joints. If invaded by wind-cold, a sense and motor disturbance may appear.

The onset of this disease is slow. The clinical manifestation is pain, which is characterized by dull pain, soreness, relieved at day and aggravated at night. More exercise during the day may activate the circulation of *qi* and blood, and relieve pain; and lying in bed at night may cause stagnation of *qi* and blood, and aggravate pain. In severe cases, inability to lift the arm, stiff joints and one-sided prominence of the acromion appear. In case of failure in treatment, heavy lifting on the healthy side will result in affection of both sides. The patient is then unable to carry out his daily activities.

Treatment:

The patient is in a sitting position with the affected shoulder exposed or with thin clothes. Examine and record the flexibility and function of the shoulder joint in order to make a comparison before and after treatment.

1) Slightly stroke the left and right shoulders, acromion, and scapula skin with the palms of both hands to relax the supraspinous muscle, deltoid muscle and scapula muscle group. The abnormal muscles are therefore exposed for treatment.

2) Grasp the muscle at the bilateral Jianjing (G 21) point with the thumbs, index fingers and middle fingers of both hands. Abnormalities, such as contracture, tightening or thickening of the muscles and tenderness, may appear at the Jianjing (G 21) point, indicating the contracture of the trapezius muscle, and stagnation of *qi* and blood. Grasping Jianjing (G 21) may relax the shoulder muscle groups and promote the circulation of *qi* and blood, thus the lifting and descending functions of the scapula muscle are improved. If the muscles fail to relax after grasping gently for a while, grasping should be done again followed by gentle percussion of the shoulders and back with the lateral palm.

3) Hold the affected wrist with one hand and lift the upper limb a little, grasp the Jiquan (H 1) and Jianzhen (SI 9) points with the other hand. After changing the hands, grasp the Jubi (Extra) and Jiquan (H 1) points to relax the muscle groups inferior and posterior to the axilla (See Fig. 3-31) and to improve the functions of the shoulder joints. A grasping maneuver may be tried on the healthy side, because in TCM there is the concept that a problem on the right side can be

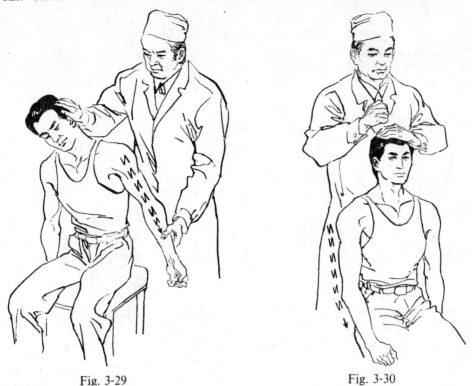

Fig. 3-29   Fig. 3-30

treated by *tuina* on left side and vice versa. The principle at work here is that the other side compensates for the problem side and so it must be treated too to bring the body back into balance.

Another method: Ask the patient to place both hands on the head. The doctor stands behind the patient and suddenly grasps the Jianzhen (SI 9) and Jiquan (H 1) points (See Fig. 3-32) with both hands or one hand when the patient is off guard. The patient said that the sudden grasping had a good effect. The abnomalities mainly appear at the deltoid muscle, teres major muscle, teres minor muscle, the broadest muscle of the back, and the infraspinous muscle superior to the armpit. Grasping these muscle groups may improve the adduction, retroflexion and internal rotation of the arm. The posterior axillary grasping stimulates the contractured muscles because the muscle contraction is under preparation.

4) Raise the affected arm level with the shoulder with one hand, press the Jianyu (LI 15) point (See Fig. 3-33) with the thumb or middle finger of another hand for a few minutes until soreness appears. Jianyu (LI 15) is located at the greater tubercle of the humerus. The common characteristic with periarthritis of the shoulder is the pain appeared at the joint between the greater tubercle of the humerus and the coracoid process. Therefore, longer pressure on this point can check the pain and improve the lifting function of the arm.

5) Pressure on the points of Quchi (LI 11), Shaohai (H 3), Shousanli (LI 10)

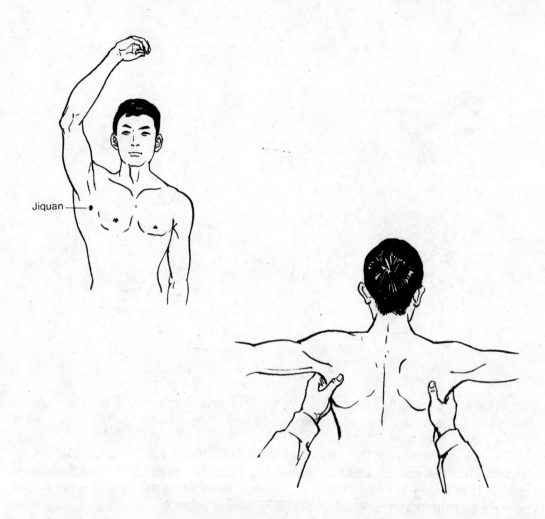

Jiquan

Fig. 3-31

and Hegu (LI 4) are applied with the fingernail.

6) Ask the patient to put his affected hand at the healthy shoulder in order to make the scapula muscle on the affected side prominent. The doctor holds the elbow behind the affected side to protrude the scapular muscle and prevent downward falling. Knead and press the points Jianjing (G 21), Bingfeng (SI 12), Tianzong (SI 11), Jianzhen (SI 9) and Ashi with the thumb gradually increasing the finger force. For periarthritis of the shoulder, contracture and pain mostly appear at this area, which is one of the factors affecting the shoulder functions. Pressing and kneading may alleviate pain and improve the functions. (See Fig. 3-34).

7) Rotate the affected arm as far as possible to the lower back. In case of

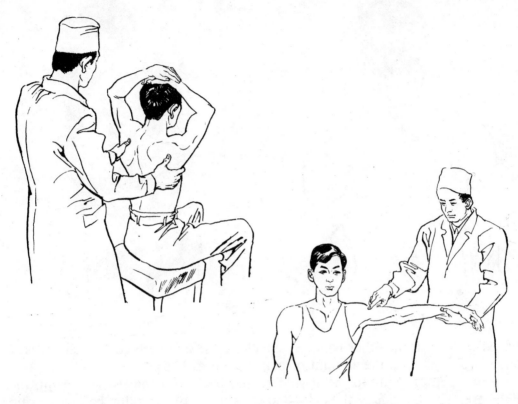

Fig. 3-32   Fig. 3-33

difficulty in rotation, try to bend the arm as much as possible. If the affected arm is only bént to the hip, support the arm with the doctor's kneecap to prevent falling. Hold the shoulder with one hand, and roll the spina scapulae, deltoid muscle, infraspinous muscle, teres major, minor muscle, and the broadest muscle of the back with the other hand (See Fig. 3-35).

8) Shaking the shoulder joints: The patient is in a sitting position and the doctor stands one meter away from the affected side with both legs apart. Hold the middle finger of the affected arm with one hand, and rotate it in a small circle (clockwise and counterclockwise alternately). Shake it suddenly when the patient is off guard (See Fig. 2-24).

9) Rolling the arm and underarm with the shoulders raised (See Figs. 2-43/44): Chat with the patient to disperse his attention, and straighten the body slowly when the patient is not aware of it. Raise the affected arm to the maximum.

10) Shaking the shoulder joints: The patient is in a sitting position and the doctor stands behind the patient. Hold the shoulder peak with one hand and the

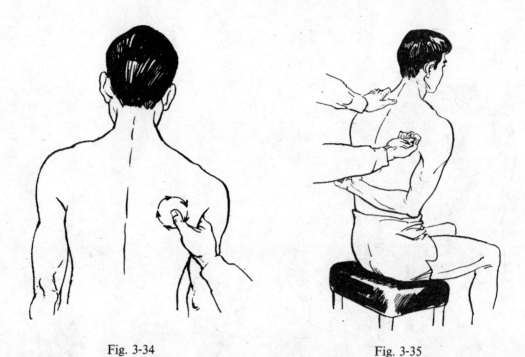

Fig. 3-34   Fig. 3-35

affected wrist with the other hand. Shake clockwise and then counterclockwise in a large circle based on the amount of pain (See Fig. 2-26).

Finally, percuss and tap the shoulders and back with the fist and palm, then tap the arm with the side of the palm and the surface of the palm, before finishing the treatment, gently stroke the shoulders, back and arm.

Typical Case:

A teacher aged 51 came to the clinic in July 1976, and complained of inability to raise his right arm, inability to rotate the forearm, inability to put his hand into his pocket, to wash his face and his hair, difficulty in taking off clothes, and pain aggravated at night for half a year, without a history of trauma. He was treated in many hospitals without improvement. Examination: prominence of the shoulder peak. Diagnosis: periarthritis of the shoulder. After being treated once with the above-mentioned method, some success was achieved. The affected arm could be lifted to 110°. The internal rotation of the shoulder was somewhat improved (from the lateral aspect of the hip to the coccyx). *Tuina* therapy was applied three times a week. After more than 10 treatments, the raising ability was close to the normal height (170°), but the prominence of the shoulder peak still remained. The internal rotation of the shoulder could reach 90°, still not reaching the scapula. After another two months treatment, the internal rotation of the shoulder was more than 90° and the prominence of the shoulder peak restored to normal. After the right side recovered, the left side was affected. After being treated for another two weeks the case was cured. No relapse was found in a follow-up visit five years later.

IV. PAIN OF THE UPPER LIMBS

1. Brachialgia

Brachialgia, divided into pain of the forearm and pain of the upper arm, occuring mostly on one side, is caused by the invasion of wind-cold, sprain, contusion and nerve injury. The clinical manifestations are dull pain and soreness. In case of injury of the ulnar nerve or radial nerve, there may appear sensory disturbance (a numb area), deformity (drop of the wrist, inability to straighten the fingers, and hand bending like a claw) and muscular atrophy.

Treatment:

For brachialgia due to invasion by wind-cold, sprain or contusion, *tuina* therapy may achieve good results, and for that due to nerve injury, provided that the nerves are not broken, *tuina* may also get good results. In general, digital pressing, kneading and grasping, picking-up, pressure with the fingernail and gentle rubbing are applied. The corresponding points with different manipulations are selected according to the various locations of the pain.

Hegu (LI 4) and Quchi (LI 11) are pressed with the fingernail in the case of pain of the forearm, and Hegu (LI 4), Shousanli (LI 10), Quchi (LI 11) and Xiaohai (SI 8) are used in case of pain of the lower part of the upper arm, and Hegu (LI 4), Quchi (LI 11), Jianyu (LI 15), the lower part of Jianyu (LI 15), Binao (LI 14), Naohui (SJ 13) and Shaohai (H 3) are chosen in case of pain of the upper part of the upper arm.

Typical Case:

A midwife aged 60 suffered from forearm pain in the summer of 1971. Analgesics failed to alleriate the problem. There was no red swelling in the examination. Hegu (LI 4) was pressed with the fingernail on the affected side for one minute and the case was cured. A follow-up visit showed no relapse.

Another male cadre aged 52 came to the clinic on November 17, 1985 and complained of a subcutaneous sharp pain on the forearm, which was unsuccessfully treated with analgesic plaster. He was unable to hold objects and had intolerable pain when wearing clothes. The cause of the pain was due to lifting heavy objects and attacks by cold. The pain lasted for several years and was recently aggravated. The treatment was performed as follows:

1) Quchi (LI 11) and Shousanli (LI 10) were pressed and kneaded as well as the subcutaneous nodules.

2) Lieque (L 7) and Waiguan (SJ 5) and the nearby subcutaneous nodules are pressed and kneaded.

3) Gently and repeatedly stroke the pain at the lateral aspect of the forearm.

The pain was basically relieved. The follow-up visits in the next year showed no relapse. Sometimes, there was mild pain, but it was cured after slight stroking and pressure for a while.

2. Numbness and Pain of the Fingers

Pain and numbness of the fingers may appear in many kinds of diseases, such as rheumatism, rheumatoid disease, disorders of the cervical vertebra, nerve injuries, contusion and spasm of the fingers. This section deals with spasm of the fingers resulting from contusion and repeated movements, which are clinically manifested as swollen pain of the finger joints, flexion impairment, and even snap-finger.

Treatment:

The treatment procedures are as follows:

1) Support the patient's hand with the palm downward and ask the patient to straighten the affected fingers. Slightly rub (See Fig. 2-17) the affected fingers centripetally with the index finger, middle finger and the ring finger forming a convex. Repeated rubbing may activate the circulation of *qi* and blood in the fingers and relieve pain.

2) With the thumb and index fingers, rotate the affected finger joints for a few minutes, first on both sides of the joints and then at the medial and lateral aspects of the joints.

3) Fix the root of the finger with one hand, and grasp the first finger knuckle or the second finger knuckle. Pull and push the fingers in order to extend the joints. A clear clicking sound may be heard. After the fingers are extended, the affected fingers feel comfortable. If the fingers fail to be stretched, the treatment can be repeated, provided that violent force is not applied, otherwise the finger ligaments may be injured.

4) After twisting and stretching, flick the back of the finger joints to dredge the meridians and collaterals.

5) Support the affected wrist with one hand, and clip the root of the affected finger with the index finger and the middle finger bending like pincers and a sudden grip is applied on both sides of the finger or on the medial and lateral sides of the finger. After gripping, the affected finger should feel comfortable. Attention should be paid to gripping neither too tightly nor too forcefully in order to prevent injuring the finger skin.

6) Slightly rub and stroke the fingers and the back of the hand before finishing the treatment.

Typical Case:

A female cadre aged 40 came to the clinic in the summer of 1973, and complained of flexion of the right little finger and inability to straighten it for many years. The finger was kneaded and rotated according to the above method for one hour. The finger was able to straighten and the patient was told the method for self-treatment to strengthen the effects.

3. Tenosynovitis

Tenosynovitis, mostly occurring at the wrist and hand, results from injury. As acute suppurative tenosynovitis caused by trauma is not a *tuina* indication, no details are introduced here. Traumatic tenosynovitis may occur at all ages, and frequently in women. This condition is ascribed to the continuous abduction of the thumb (such as carrying a baby and twisting clothes) and a long period of holding a hard object in the hand (such as holding scissors, ironing clothes and holding cooking utensils). The clinical manifestations are difficulty in abduction of the thumb, pain, slight swelling of the styloid process of the radius associated with tenderness, and severe pain at the styloid process of the radius when the thumb is in adduction, when making a fist and at the same time moving laterally. Therefore, the patient with this case has difficulties in holding objects.

Treatment:

Traumatic tenosynovitis may be treated either by an operation or by *tuina* therapy. The points Lieque (L 7), Hegu (LI 4), Yangxi (LI 5), Yangchi (SJ 4), Waiguan (SJ 5), Quze (P 3) and Jianzhen (SI 9) are often selected. First, apply slight stroking, then pressing, kneading, pushing and grasping. Slight stroking may relieve the pain, while pressing and kneading may soften and minimize the hard protuberances. A small protuberance often occurs at the dorsal aspect of the wrist and is sunk into the bone space during pressing. The wrist should be placed in such a position that the small protuberance cannot be moved away when pressing and kneading are performed. The force should be from light to heavy and talcum powder should be used to prevent injuring the skin. Each pressing and kneading may relieve the pain and soften and reduce the vesicular protuberance. Push the vesicular protuberance with the thumb crease upward more and downward less. Or ask the patient to raise his arm high, and then push the vesicular protuberance at the dorsum of the hand and wrist from above to below, and at the same time, heavily grasp the underarm.

Typical Case:

A woman violinist aged 28 suffered from tenosynovitis of the left hand associated with severe pain because of playing the violin frequently. After being treated 13 times (every other day) with the above method, the case was basically cured.

V. HYPERTENSION

Hypertension, a commonly encountered disease, is considered to be within the range of dizziness and headache in traditional Chinese medicine. This case often takes place in the elderly. The clinical manifestations include the increase of arterial pressure, headache, dizziness, head distension, flushed face and hot temper. Chinese medicine ascribes this condition to the disturbance of *yin* and *yang* in the liver and kidney.

Tuina is certainly effective in treating hypertension at the initial and intermediate stages, but not satisfactory for hypertension at the later period. *Tuina* is not permitted when there has been a cerebrosascular accident, especially at its acute phase. *Tuina* therapy may be related to the manipulations and the functions on the meridians and acupoints, which may relax exmotional tension, regulate the equilibrium of *qi*, blood, *yin* and *yang* and lower the blood pressure. *Tuina* treatment on the chest, back, abdomen and the four limbs may relieve the spasm of the general fine arteries, reduce the peripheral resistance and lower the blood pressure.

Treatment:

1) Apply *tuina* on the points of the Bladder Meridian and Du Meridian:

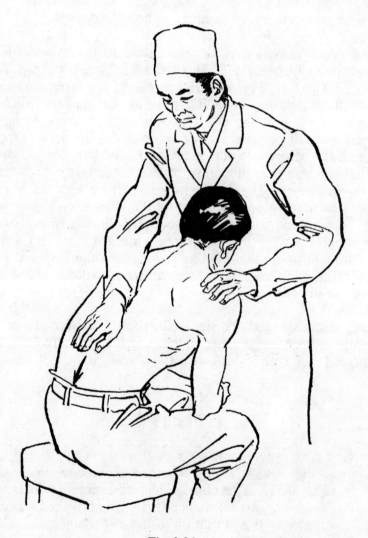

Fig. 3-36

A. The patient is in a sitting position with the head bent forward to expose the back, lower back and buttock completely, while the doctor stands in front of the patient's head. Gently and forcefully push the spine and with the palm from above to below (See Fig. 3-36). Horizontally push the Bladder Meridian on both sides of the spine medially from the Fengmen (B 12) to Baihuanshu (B 30) points and laterally from Fufen (B 4) to Zhibian (B 54) for 3-5 or 5-7 times respectively, and then push the Du Meridian from the Dazhui (Du 14) to Changqiang (Du 1) points 3-5 or 5-7 times. After the pushing is finished on the back, the skin will have five red lines.

B. Grasping, lifting and releasing are respectively performed in the orders of A along the *Du* Meridian (one line) and the Bladder Meridian (two lines). After grasping, five red lines should appear on the skin surface of the back.

C. Press the points (every other finger width) with the thumb on the above-mentioned five lines from above to below 3-5 or 5-7 times. The finger force should be from light to heavy and vice versa. For example, if pressing for five times, the first time is light, the second time a little heavier, the third time heavier, the fourth time light and the fifth time lighter. After pressing, five red dotted lines appeared on the back.

D. Press along the five lines with the thenar for the same number of times. The finger force exerted is the same as that mentioned above. After grasping is applied, the dotted red lines are connected in a patch shape.

E. Press the Mingmen (Du 4), Yaoyangguan (Du 3), Yaoshu (Du 2), Changqiang (Du 1), Sanjiaoshu (B 22), Shenshu (B 23), Qihaishu (B 24), Dachangshu (B 25), Xiaochangshu (B 27), Baihuanshu (B 30), Huangmen (B 51), Zhibian (B 54) and Baliao (B 31-34) points with the thumb of both hands. The key point for force exertion: a little heavier than the digital pressing, but the force should be gradually increased and reduced. Heavy force should not be used when beginning the pressure. A test strength should be tried in the first pressing so that the patient is able to develop tolerance.

F. Percuss, tap and beat the above-mentioned lines several times with the fist, palm and lateral palm.

G. Slightly stroke the back and lower back with the extended palm several times before finishing the treatment. The function of the manipulation is to strengthen the kidney. The clinical experiments have proved effective in lowering blood pressure. In general, after a few treatments the systolic pressure can drop by 10 mm Hg in comparison before and after *tuina*.

2) Rest for a while, and then apply the following manipulations:

A. The patient is still in a prone position and the doctor stands behind the patient's buttock. Push horizontally with one palm along the running course of the Bladder Meridian posterior to the left lower limb from the Chengfu (B 36) to Pushen (B 61) points 3-5 or 5-7 times, and then do the same on the right side.

B. Push along both sides of the lower limb with palms of both hands from the root of the leg to both sides of the malleolus 3-5 or 5-7 times.

C. Roll the posterior aspect of the lower limb. The starting and ending points and the rolling times are the same.

D. Grasp the muscles on both sides of the lower limb with one hand, advancing from the root of the leg to the Kunlun (B 60) point and then vice versa several times.

E. Press the points of Chengfu (B 36), Yinmen (B 37), Weizhong (B 40), Weiyang (B 39), Chengshan (B 57) and Fengshi (B 31) with the thumb. Grasp the Kunlun (B 60) point and rub the Yongquan (K 1) point for the same length of time as mentioned before.

F. Percussing, tapping and beating are applied with light to heavy force and vice versa several times with the fist, palm, the finger tips and the lateral palm before the treatment is finished.

The function of the manipulation is to dredge the meridians and collaterals of the lower limbs, dilate the fine arteries of the lower limbs, reduce the peripheral resistance and activate the blood circulation to lower the blood pressure.

3) *Tuina* manipulations on the chest and abdomen:

A. The patient is in a supine position with the chest and abdomen exposed. Massage the Tanzhong (Ren 17) point with the palm of the thumb or the middle finger for two minutes, then massage the Zhongwan (Ren 12), Jianli (Ren 11) and Qihai (Ren 6) points respectively for two minutes (See Figs. 3-37/38), and then slightly stroke (or push) from the Tanzhong (Ren 17) to Qihai (Ren 6) points five times, which function to soothe the chest oppression and benefit the diaphragm, to drop the upward liver *qi* and to induce *qi* to come back to Qihai (Ren 6). Tanzhong (Ren 17) is a *qi* point. In case of depression and belching, the patient will feel comfortable after massaging this point. Press the points Zhongwan (Ren 12), Jianli (Ren 11) and Qihai (Ren 6) to induce *qi* to descend, then slight stroking (or pushing) is applied to help *qi* come back to the original Qihai (Ren 6) point.

B. The position remains the same and the operator stands on the right side of the patient. Push horizontally from the external aspect of the right nipple to the external aspect of the left nipple (Tanzhong Ren 17 is located between the nipples) with the left palm, and at the same time, push from the left side of the umbilicus to the right side of the umbilicus with the right palm five times (See Fig. 3-39). The continuous left and right pushing is able to regulate the horizontally attacked liver *qi*.

C. Palm-rubbing along the intercostal nerve from the underarm to the umbilicus for more than five times (See Fig. 3-40).

D. Knead and rub the abdomen when the patient is in a supine position:

i) Slowly rub around the umbilicus clockwise with one hand for three minutes.

ii) Roll the abdomen in all directions with one hand for three minutes.

iii) Knead and push the umbilicus with either the separating or joining maneuver for two minutes.

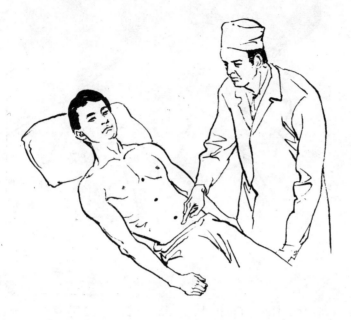

Fig. 3-37

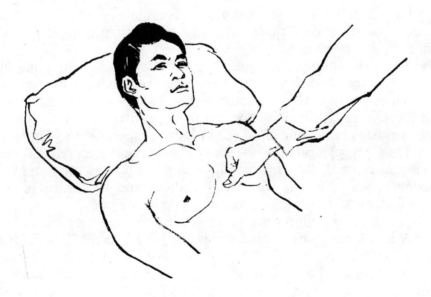

Fig. 3-38

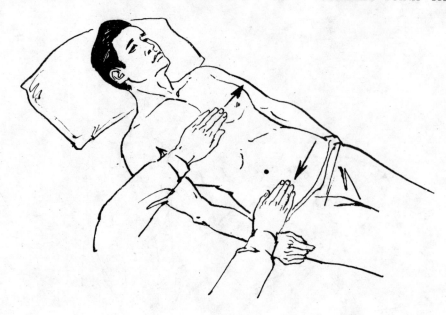

Fig. 3-39

iv) Knead and press the Jianli (Ren 11), Liangmen (S 21), Zhangmen (Liv 13), Youmen (K 21), Qihai (Ren 6), and Guanyuan (Ren 4) points with the index finger, the middle finger and the ring finger of one hand for five minutes. Right Liangmen (S 21) and left Zhangmen (Liv 13) may be kneaded and pressed for a longer time. In case of a delicate constitution, the Qihai (Ren 6) and Guanyuan (Ren 4) points should be kneaded and presses for a longer time.

v) Percuss the abdomen with the lateral palm and slightly stroke the abdomen before finishing the treatment.

Rubbing and kneading the abdomen are very important in treating hypertension and some complicated chronic internal diseases though the mechanism is still not clear. Important organs are located in the abdomen. The umbilicus, which relates to the five zang organs, is located in the centre of the abdomen. Many important meridians also gathered in the abdomen, especially the Chong and Ren meridians. The Chong Meridian is the sea of the 12 regular meridians and the Du Meridian is the sea of all the *yang* meridians. Since a part of the Ren Meridian is in the abdomen and connects with the umbilicus and the heart, pressing and rubbing the abdomen helps regulate *yin* and *yang* in the body.

The above three procedures are all effective for hypertension, and are used alternately or in combination, which depends upon the time required for treatment.

Typical Case:

A male engineer aged 58 had hypertension for 14 years. Daily medication of both Chinese herbs and verticils could not stop the increasing blood pressure. Headache, dizziness and muscle pain were daily aggravated, and his blood pressure

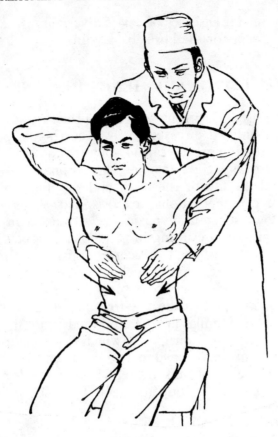

Fig. 3-40

reached 200/130 mm Hg. The subcutaneous muscle of the lower limbs was hard and painful. The patient received *tuina* treatment on October 28, 1986 and felt better after one treatment. Then the medication was stopped. After six continuous treatments, the blood pressure dropped to 170/100 mm Hg. After 14 treatments, it dropped to 164/100 mm Hg, and after 21 treatments, it dropped to 170/90 mm Hg. From that time on, the blood pressure remained normal. Because of excessive drinking at Spring Festival, the blood pressure was a little elevated and then dropped to 160/90 mm Hg. headache, dizziness, and pain of the lower limbs were basically relieved and the hardness in the muscle disappeared.

A male chief engineer aged 59 had hypertension for 20 years. The pathological condition was intermittent after being treated in some hospitals and medication of Chinese herbs and verticils. He came to the clinic on November 10, 1986 and the blood pressure at that time was 170/100 mm Hg, accompanied by headache, dizziness, disease of the cervical vertebra and lower back pain. After *tuina* treatment, there was some improvement. After a course of treatment, the blood pressure dropped to 140/90 mm Hg, and after more treatments, the blood pressure remained at 130/80 mm Hg. Diseases of cervical vertebra, headache and dizziness were basically cured except for the lower back pain.

VI. CORONARY HEART DISEASE

Coronary heart disease, i.e., coronary ateriosclerotic cardiopathy, is a commonly and frequently encountered disease mostly occurring in people over 40. The number of cases is increasing every year, in younger and younger people and it is especially common in over weight people. The coronary arteries are the blood vessels curving around the top of the heart and supplying blood to the cardiac muscles. In the case of athermatous sclerosis, narrowing of the lumen and reduction of blood flow, ischemia, hypoxia and arteriospasm take place to some extent in the cardiac muscles, resulting in metabolic products such as lactic acid and phosphoric acid, which give rise to precordium pain by stimulating the nerves. In mild cases precordium depression or a slight stabbing pain may appear, while in severe cases, angina pectoris may occur for a few seconds to a few minutes. If angina pectoris continues, the heartbeat is irregula, contraction is weak and the blood pressure drops. Arrhythmia, heart failure and acute myocardiac infarction due to cardiogenic shock may be considered, which is the main factor for a sudden death. All these symptoms may be due to overstraining, forceful exertion in holding breath, carrying heavy objects, overeating, excessive drinking or too much smoking, emotional excitement, sudden attack by cold or heat, or intake of excessive greasy food.

Treatment:

1) According to different conditions of patients, psychotherapy should be first given to confirm the patient's confidence in the treatment, such as the introduction of the principle of treatment or the past treatment methods. The digital rubbing of Ashi points is performed on the chest with the middle finger, and the patient is asked to put his left palm on the left side of the chest and to rhythmically percuss the dorsum of the left hand with his right loosened fist in order to dilate the contractured blood vessels and relieve the pain.

2) Massage the Ren and Chong meridians on the chest and abdomen to regulate the *qi* flow and activate the blood circulation when the patient is in a supine position. The manipulations are similar to items A, B, and C (in 1) for hemiplegia. Then massage, roll and rub the anterior and lateral aspects of the lower limbs for about 10 minutes.

3) When the patient is in a prone position, press, rub, pick up, knead, push and roll the Bladder Meridian and Du Meridian with procedures similar with those (A-G in 1) for hypertension. Afterward, massage the posterior aspect of the lower limbs for about 10 minutes.

Typical Case:

A woman doctor aged 55 suffered from coronary heart disease in recent years, accompanied by precordium depression, stabbing pain and attacks of angina pectoris. On July 1, 1984, she received the first treatment with routine procedures as mentioned above. Since the patient had a weak constitution, gentle manipulation with both reinforcing and reduing was applied. After the treatment, the depression was relieved. Then the patient continued the treatment, and had a massaage once a day, 20 minutes each. Sixteen treatments in all were given, and the case was basically cured. The patient is still healthy and is able to go swimming.

VII. HEMIPLEGIA

Hemiplegia refers to the motor failure (complete paralysis) or motor limit (incomplete paralysis) on either side of the upper or lower limbs, and is a sequela mostly resulting from windstroke. *Tuina* therapy has traditionally been used in China to treat hemplegia. As recorded in the Internal Classics, "obstruction of the meridians and collacterals may result in numbness, which can be treated by massage." Clinical practice has proven that the functions could be mostly recovered in mild cases and patients were able to walk with the help of a cane in case of immediate massage treatment. For severe cases, some functions can be restored and the patient can carry out his daily activities. Therefore, *tuina* therapy is an auxillary method for treating sequela of cerebral accident. However, those with severe pathological conditions, loss of consciousness and failing to cooperate are not advised to have *tuina* treatment.

Treatment:

Prior to treatment, the pathological conditions should be inquired about by means of inspection, auscultation, interrogation and palpitation, such as the degree of hemiplegia, weakness or spasm of the joints, muscles and tendons, location of pain and numbness, excess or deficiency type of constitution and the complications. In general, pushing, rolling, pressing, grasping, twisting, gripping, rubbing, rotating, shaking and stroking are frequently applied on the chest, abdomen, the upper and lower limbs, lower back, back, head and face.

The *tuina* sequence is as follows:

1) The patient is in a supine position and the doctor stands on the right side of the patient.

A. Slightly stroke from the point Xuanji (Ren 21) to the point Qihai (Ren 6) with the palm of one hand several times.

B. Press and knead the Tanzhong (Ren 17), Juque (Ren 14), Zhongwan (Ren 12), Jianli (Ren 11) and Qihai (Ren 6) points with either the thumb or the middle finger of one hand.

C. Horizontally push from right to left along the line of left and right Ruzhong (S 17) and Tanzhong (Ren 17) points on the chest, and along the line of the Shenque (Ren 8), Huangshu (K 16), Tianshu (S 25) and Daheng (Sp 15) points on the abdomen, then rub from left to right via the abdoman (basically similar as with hypertension) for three minutes. The function is to remove the stagnation from the chest, benefit the diaphragm and to regulate the horizontally attacked liver *qi*.

2) *Tuina* on the affected upper limb with one hand:

A. Raise the affected upper limb and gently stroke from above to below with one hand several times.

B. Hold the affected arm with one hand, grasp and pick up the muscles of one side of the upper limb from above to below alternating the hands.

C. Hold the affected limb with one hand, and press the Jianyu (LI 15), Binao (LI 14), Jugu (LI 16), Qugu (Ren 2), Shaohai (H 3), Chize (L 5), Shousanli (LI 10) and Hegu (LI 4) points with either the thumb or the middle finger of the other hand.

D. Move the wrist with one hand and knead, press, grasp and pick up the Yangxi (LI 5), Yanggu (SI 5), Yangchi (SJ 4), Zhongquan (Extra 25), Daling (P 7), Taiyuan (L 9), Shenmen (H 7), Neiguan (P 6) and Waiguan (SJ 5) points with the other hand.

E. Hold the affected fingers with one hand, and gently rub, twist, knead, flick and grip the affected fingers with the other hand for five minutes.

3) Remove trousers to expose the affected leg for application of *tuina*:

A. Horizontally push the leg (anterior and both sides) from above to below several times.

B. Either press with the fingernail, or grasp Qichong (S 30), Maibu (Extra), Futu(S 32), Zusanli (S 36), Jiexi (S 41), Chongmen (Sp 12), Jimen (Sp 11), Xuehai (Sp 10), Yanglingquan (G 34), Sanyinjiao (Sp 6) and Taichong (Liv 3) points with the thumb.

C. Progressively grasp the muscles of both sides of the leg from below to above (See Fig. 3-41).

D. Percuss, tap and puncture the anterior and both sides of the leg respectively with the fist, palm, lateral palm and with the fingers closed.

E. Gentle stroking is applied several times, 5-7 minutes each before finishing the treatment.

4) When the patient is in a prone position, apply *tuina* with the routine chiropractic on the back and lower back, with the emphasis on pressing the Ganshu (B 18), Shenshu (B 23), Yaoyangguan (Du 3) and Mingmen (Du 4) points for five minutes.

5) *Tuina* on the posterior aspect of the lower limbs:

A. Horizontally push from above to below several times.

B. Press with the thumb the points Huantiao (G 30), Qianjin, Fengshi (G 31), Xuanzhong (G 39), Zhibian (B 54), Chengfu (B 36), Weizhong (B 40), Weiyang (B 39), Chengjin (B 56), Chengshan (B 57), Kunlun (B 60), Shenmai (B 62) and Jinmen (B 63).

C. Roll the muscles on the posterior aspect of the lower limb, emphasizing the popliteal fossa.

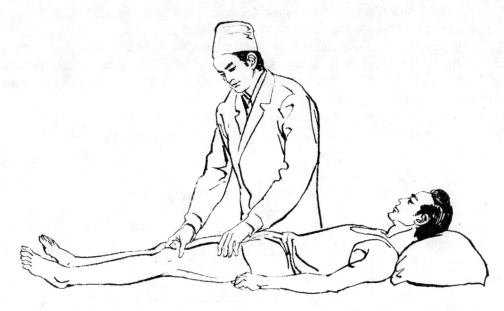

Fig. 3-41

D. Percuss with the fist and palm.

E. Gently stroke for five minutes.

The above-mentioned procedures may be selected according to the pathological condition. Simple manipulation may be done on the healthy side. Generally, treat for 15-30 minutes each time.

Forceful manipulation should not be used on a stiff elbow or wrist, and in flexion disturbance. *Tuina* is applied patiently. If one treatment is not enough, more treatments are required to gradually restore the functions.

Typical Case:

The methods for treating hemiplegia are many, but the whole process of treatment is not necessary. After recovery, the patient is advised to do exercises. For example, some male patients from ages 54-82 had hemiplegia from half a year to 18 years. The symptoms are hemiparalysis (one leg or one arm), inability to roll, to sit and to walk, and inability to speak and dementia. Those with mild conditions could walk with the help of a stick or other people. Having been treated according to the above procedures 1), 2) and 3), good results were obtained. Some could roll over, walk with the support of a stick or the wall, and most of the patients could walk without any help. Satisfactory results were not achieved however in the case of spasm of the forearm and stiff fingers.

A male aged 70 had hemiparalysis for 16 years. He had fallen down three times in recent years, and the condition worsened after each fall. After was treated with *tuina* therapy twice, he could walk again.

A patient had hemiplegia after windstroke. He was unable to roll over, sit and walk. After being treated three times, he could roll over, sit and walk holding the wall. After more treatments, he could walk freely.

A male aged 75 was admitted to the hospital three times for emergency treatment after windstroke. He could not speak but could take small steps with the help of a stick. After two massage treatments, he could walk with large steps and go up and down stairs supported by others.

Patients under 60 may achieve better results. After several *tuina* treatments, they could walk with the help of stick and could walk normally after doing some exercises.

VIII. ABDOMINAL DISORDERS

1. Stomach Pain

Stomach pain, also known as epigastric pain, is a common problem. Chinese medicine holds that stomach pain results from failure of stomach *qi* to descend, which may arise from melancholy, anger and depression of liver *qi* encroaching upon the stomach, or may occur when the depression of *qi* is transformed into fire which attacks the stomach. It may also be due to stagnation of *qi* and blood stasis. Other etiological factors include weakness of stomach *qi* associated with invasion of cold, insufficient *yang qi* leading to internal cold, thus resulting in condensation of cold and stagnation of *qi*, and excessive eating of raw and cold food, and abnormal eating which injure the spleen and stomach, leading to the failure of stomach *qi* to descend. The etiology should be analyzed according to the symptoms and treatment is administered based on differentiation.

Treatment:

1) Pain due to cold in the stomach mostly results from deficiency-cold in the spleen and stomach and there is dull pain which may be relieved by warmth and pressure. The procedures are as follows:

A. The patient is in a supine position. Rub the epigastric region slowly with the palm for five minutes in order to penetrate the warm *qi* into the stomach, warm the middle *jiao* to dispel cold and normalizing the stomach function to alleviate the pain (See Fig. 3-42). After the above procedure is performed, the pain is mostly relieved. In case of severe pain, after rubbing slowly for a while, press the epigastric region with three fingers or with the palm in combination with pressing the points of Jianjing (G 21), Tanzhong (Ren 17), Zusanli (S 36), Hegu (LI 4), Neiguan (P 6), Qimen (Liv 14), Zhangmen (Liv 13) and Qihai (Ren 6). The separating and joining maneuvers are also applied to the epigastric region. Percuss the abdomen with the lateral palm followed by light stroking before the treatment is finished.

B. When the patient is in a prone position, either a stroking or horizontal pushing maneuver is applied on the points of the Bladder Meridian on both sides of the spine, with the emphasis on pressing Ganshu (B 18), Weishu (B 21), Pishu (B 20) and Sanjiaoshu (B 22) with heavy force 3-5 times, then percussion, striking

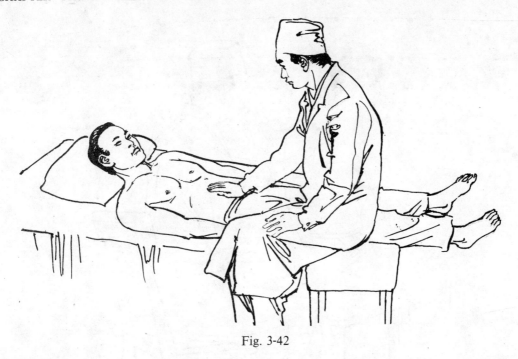

Fig. 3-42

and light stroking are performed five minutes before the treatment is finished.

Typical Case:

A women peasant of 65 years old had general stomach pain. During the attack, the pain was severe and could be relieved after taking analgesics. One day in late autumn of 1971, she had a sudden attack with strong pain. Massage with the above procedures was done for 15 minutes and then the pain was relieved. The patient remained healthy in the follow-up visits over a period of five years.

2) Pain due to retention of food:

This condition results from over eating and drinking which injures the spleen and stomach leading to retention of food. The manifestations include distending pain of the epigastric region, which is resistant to pressure, and aggravated after eating, belching and sour regurgitation. The *tuina* method is as follows (No massage should be done in case of overeating or fasting):

A. Take a sitting position and massage the points of the Bladder Meridian on both sides of the spine from the point Dazhui (Du 14) to the point Mingmen (Du 4), then press and knead Gaohuang (B 43), Weishu (B 21), Pishu (B 20), Shenshu (B 23) and Sanjiaoshu (B 22). Then tap and percuss both sides of the spine with the fist or the palm (See Fig. 3-43).

B. Massage the stomach region with one hand, i.e. palm-rubbing, the stomach from the cardia to the pylorus. Palm-rubbing in the opposite direction is seldom used. This method strengthens the peristalsis of the stomach, strengthens digestion and absorption, removes retention in the stomach, activates the flow of stomach

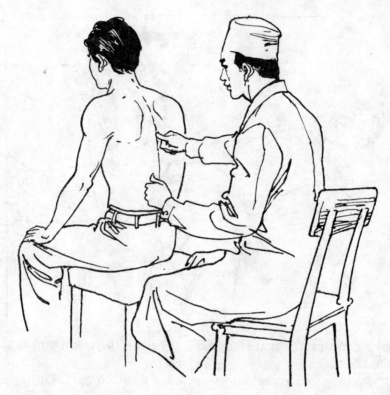

Fig. 3-43

qi and relieves distending epigastric pain and fullness.

3) Pain due to liver *qi* attacking the stomach.

This condition mostly arises from anger and emotional frustration leading to depression of liver *qi*. In the case of long standing depression of liver *qi*, the liver *qi* will travel upward or horizontally and attack the spleen and stomach, resulting in the failure of stomach *qi* to descend and epigastric pain. Clinical manifestations are distending pain in the upper abdomen, often radiating to the chest, costal region, and back, and frequent belching. In addition, there may be loss of appetite, listlessness and weakness in the limbs. These symptoms are similar to gastrointestinal neurosis in Western medicine. The principle of treatment is to regulate the *qi* flow of the liver and normalize the stomach. The *tuina* procedure is as follows:

A. Apply *tuina* on the Bladder Meridian on the back with the same manipulations as mentioned before. First grasp the Jianjing (G 21) point, then digitally press the Gaohuang (B 43), Ganshu (B 18), Weishu (B 21), Pishu(B 20) and Shenshu (B 23) points. The functions of the Zang-Fu organs are regulated through the therapeutic function of the Shu points, and also through the strengthening of kidney water to restrain liver wood, seeking to treat both the root cause and the symptoms and relieving pain by soothing the liver and normalizing the stomach.

B. Apply *tuina* on the chest and abdomen, press and knead in sequence the Tanzhong (Ren 17), Liangmen (S 21), Zhongwan (Ren 12), Tianshu (S 25), Qihai (Ren 6), Qimen (Liv 14) and Zhangmen (Liv 13) points. Gently push from the point Tanzhong (Ren 17) to Qihai (Ren 6) continuously several times, then obliquely push with both hands from both subaxillae of the left and right intercostal regions and further to the umbilicus and abdomen. The function is to remove the stagnation of *qi* in the upper abdomen, soothe the liver and regulate *qi* flow, send abnormally ascending *qi* down and check pain. Then push horizontally on the left and right at the space between Tanzhong (Ren 17) and Liangmen (S 21), and at the space between the Shenque (Ren 8) and Qihai (Ren 6). (i.e., horizontal pushing from right to left at the chest and that from left to right at the umbilicus, do not push to and fro at the same place). The difference from the previous procedure on the chest and abdomen is the adding to the points Liangmen (S 21), Zhangmen (Liv 13) and Qimen (Liv 14). Knead and press the right Liangmen (S 21) point mainly with the reinforcing method.

Typical Case:

A male doctor aged 73 was admitted to the hospital in spring, 1981 because of abdominal pain. He stayed in the hospital for about five months and was greated with 50-60 decoctions of Chinese herbs. The pain was relieved but not eliminated. Intermittent pain attacked every day for about five hours. Examination showed free of positive signs and the etiology was not clear. Several doctors were consulted and the diagnosis tended to the injury of gastric muscosa and gastrointestinal neurosis. Massage was done once every day according to the above-mentioned method. The pain was greatly relieved and the pain was reduced from five to two hours after 1-2 *tuina* treatments, and pain disappeared after another four treatments. The patient rested for a few days during the treatment and felt a little uncomfortable but no relapse occurred. Thirteen *tuina* treatments in all cured the case.

2. Abdominal Pain:

Abdominal pain, a commonly encountered symptom may appear in many diseases. Therefore, its etiology is very complicated, relating to internal, gynecological and pediatric disorders. Abdominal pain arises from invasion of cold, and retention of food and may be treated by *tuina* therapy. However *tuina* therapy is contraindicated in cases of acute abdominal pain resulting from intestinal perforation and obstruction, rupture or infarction of the parenchymatous organs, biliary calculi and ureterolith. The details of the case history and a careful examination should be made for patients with abdominal pain, in which the former includes asking the location, acute or chronic and period of abdominal pain; nature of pain; the time of abdominal pain; and complications. In general, pain around the umbilicus with a long course, chronic onset, dull pain, turning pain or vague pain is an indication for *tuina* therapy, while severe pain which may be relieved by warmth and pressure is the contraindication provided that the test strength is applied. Since pathological conditions of abdominal pain are very ocmplicated, especially for acute abodominal pain the masseur should be very careful in the treatment. Abdominal pain with an acute onset should be managed in the hospital, while that with frequent attacks and a confirmed hospital diagnosis may be treated with *tuina* therapy.

Treatment:

1) Massage the back, abdomen and legs. According to the principle that "in emergency cases treat the acute symptoms first, when these are relieved, treat the root cause." Pushing, digital pressing, lifting, rubbing, tapping, percussing, beating and stroking maneuvers are first applied on the Bladder Meridian of the back, with emphasis on pressing the points Pishu (B 20), Weishu (B 21), Dachangshu (B 25), Xiaochangshu (B 27), Weizhong (B 40) and Chengshan (B 57), which may enhance the pain-resisting ability of the whole body, relieve abdominal pain and set up the conditions for massage of the abdomen.

2) For intolerable abdominal pain suitable for *tuina* treatment the abdomen may first be massaged. The patient is asked to take a supine position with the abdomen exposed, and the doctor sits besides the patient.

A. Rub the umbilicus and its surrounding area slowly with the palm of one hand for five minutes. (Clockwise rubbing is mostly used for deficiency-cold syndrome).

B. Relay rubbing is done around the umbilicus with the palms of both hands for three minutes.

C. Slightly roll around the umbilicus with one hand for two minutes.

D. Knead slowly from the upper abdomen to the lower abdomen, from the right upper abdomen to the left lower abdomen and from the left upper abdomen to the right lower abdomen with the palm of one hand for three minutes.

E. Push and knead from the umbilicus in the four directions by the separating method and then from the four directions to the umbilicus by the joining method with the palms of both hands for two minutes.

F. Grasp the abdominal muscle and horizontally push from the upper abdomen to the lower abdomen for two minutes.

G. Press the Zhongwan (Ren 12), Jianli (Ren 11), Qihai (ren 6), Guanyuan (Ren 4) and Tianshu (S 25) points with the index, middle and ring fingers, press the points Liangmen (S 21), Zusanli (S 36) and Sanyinjiao (Sp 6) with the thumb, and finally best with the lateral palm and slightly stroke the abdomen before finishing the treatment. If the pathological conditions are not complicated, some maneuvers (kneading in any direction) may be reduced. Spasmotic pain of the umbilicus and abdomen may be relieved by pressure. Press continuously with one palm or overlapped palms for 3-5 minutes. Please note that heavy force should not be used. Massage is generally forbidden for excess-type abdominal pain resistant to pressing.

3. Gastroptosis

Gastroptosis, known as stomach deficiency in traditional Chinese medicine, is a commonly encountered disease, which is classified into the asthenic type, the epigastric umbilicate type and the hypogastric expansive type. The patient often has abodminal pain, abdominal distension, a bearing-down feeling in the abdomen, often accompanied by loss of appetite, mild pain occurring during eating, pain aggravated after eating, splashing sound in the lower abdomen after eating porridge food, bowel movement once every 2-3 days, constipation or diarrhea, profuse clear and frequent urine, weak limbs, dizziness, palpitation, and insomnia. A barium examination showed that at the lower border of the stomach five cm exceeded the connecting line of the illiac crest. *Tuina* therapy may achieve results.

Treatment:

1) When the patient is in a prone position, the doctor applies massage on the Du Meridian and Bladder Meridian bilaterally with manipulations similar to the routine chiropractic introduced before. Pressing, picking-up and lifting maneuvers should be emphasized on the points Geshu (B 17), Weishu (B 21) and Shenshu (B 23). In addition, concentrically horizontal pushing is applied from the sacral vertebra to the first lumbar vertebra for five minutes.

2) Press and knead the Baihui (Du 20) point with the thumb for one minute. The doctor puts his hand on the patient's shoulder joint on one side and rotates the patient's upper arm backward with the patient's forearm placed on the lower back to relax the scapular muscle. The doctor closes his five fingers of the other

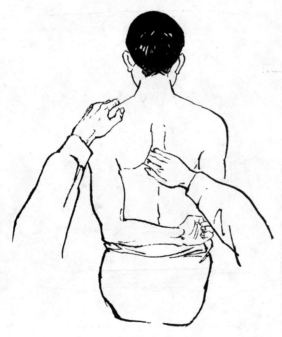

Fig. 3-44

hand and puts it at the medial margin of the midpoint (about the location of Gaohuang, B 43) of the scapula and then inserts his hand into the scapula seam obliquely superior to the acromion (See Fig. 3-44).

Main points: Press internally with one hand holding the acromion and insert the closed five fingers of the other hand slowly into the scapula seam, about 2-3 cm deep. After insertion, stay there for a while and then remove it. The patient will not feel any pain, but the descended stomach can be lifted.

3) The patient should be in a supine position with the knees flexed and the hip elevated by a pad underneath. The doctor holds the lower limb of one side for knee-chest rotatory pressing with one hand placed on the knee joint and another hand at the dorsum of the foot (See Fig. 3-45). Repeat the procedure several times on both sides. Each time the rotatory pressure should be held for a while. Then both lower limbs are raised for rotatory pressing and left there for a moment.

4) The patient should be in a supine position with the knees flexed. Lower the trousers to the hip to expose the lower abdomen (the abdominal muscle relaxed). Make both hands into fists and slightly flex the elbow, leaving a space half a *chi* wide between the two fists like a bracket. Raise both fists slowly from the lower

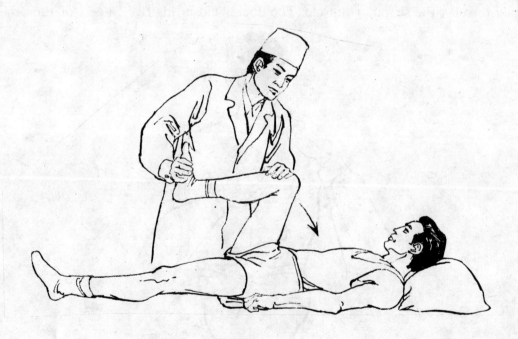

Fig. 3-45

abdomen over the head or the space between the two fists is expanded from half a *chi* to two *chi* close and open the hands in front of the chest repeatedly several times (See Fig. 4-46). At the same times, the doctor closes his five fingers and puts it on the left side below the umbilicus. The descended stomach bottom will be slowly lifted upward to the original place when the patient is doing bracket lifting or abduction so that the movement of the upper limbs, the enlargement of the chest and the lifting of the diaphram will contract the descended stomach. If the abdominal wall is not soft enough and the descended stomach bottom is felt with difficulty with the deep slippery palpation, put the stomach back to the original place with the ulnar sides of the hands pushing upward from the left and right circle sides of the abdomen.

5) Grasp, roll and knead the abdominal muscles with the five fingers of both hands in order to strengthen the contractility of the straight muscle, transverse muscle, internal oblique muscle and external oblique muscle of the abdomen. The grasping is directed from the umbilicus to the four sides, i.e. pull up and put down repeatedly. Then roll the abdominal muscle with the palm. The straight muscle is rolled from above to below and the other muscles are rolled around the umbilicus. Slight tapping with the lateral palm is applied before finishing the treatment.

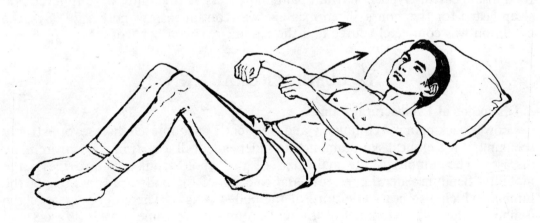

Fig. 3-46

6) Grasp the soft part of the lumbus with both hands and move the fingers when grasping from the superior margin of the iliac crest to the inferior margin of the hypochondrium. Or after grasping the soft part of the lumbus, push jointly towards the umbilicus to strengthen the contractility of the internal and external oblique muscles of the abdomen and the lumbar fascia so that the contraction of the abdominal cavity will be harmful to the ptosis of the stomach.

7) The patient is advised to strengthen the movement of the abdominal muscle, such as lifting the leg held straight, holding the knees close to the chest, semicircle raising and abduction with the upper arm adducted and the elbow flexed. At the same time, knee flexion is combined.

The above manipulations and movements are certainly effective to retract the descended stomach. If the patient is able to persist in the treatment, the appetite, can be improved, pain relieved and the stomach gradually lifted.

Typical Case:

A woman cadre aged 60 came to the clinic on September 23, 1983. Chief complaints: five cm gastroptosis, bearing down feeling in the stomach, loss of appetite, abdominal distension after eating, lassitude, pain of the hypochondrium, loose stools, scanty and dark yellow urine, enlargement of the liver, dizziness, palpitation, insomnia and excessive dreaming. She took Chinese herbs and Western drugs for several years, but obtained no marked effects. The patient was thin, and the pulse was deep, string-taut and thready. Diagnosis: gastroptosis due to depression of liver *qi* and a weak spleen. Having been treated with the above procedures seven times, the patient felt comfortable, slept well and had a better appetite. Ten *tuina* treatments were applied and the abdominal distension and bearing down feeling were greatly relieved. Originally, the abdomen was in the shape of a ship and the centre was depressed when the patient was in a supine position. After the treatments the abdomen became flat. The splashing sound after eating some dilute food disappeared. Hypochondrium pain and excessive dreaming were relieved and sleep lasted for five hours. Then massage was continued for another 20 days, the condition was completely cured and the patient resumed her work.

IX. LUMBOCRURAL PAIN

1. Discussion of Lumbocrural Pain

Lower back pain is a commonly and frequently encountered disease, but strictly speaking, it is a clinical symptom, not an independent illness. It may occur in many diseases. The lumbus is the main axis of the whole trunk and provides large mobility. Bending, lateral curvature and rotation of the body are functions of the lumbus, which also bears one third of the body's weight. The anterior part of the lumbus is the soft abdominal cavity and around it are some muscles, fascia and ligaments, but free from protection of the body structure. Therefore, in case of overloading, improper labour or movement, or a long period of an improper position, there may be injuries to the lumbar muscles, tendons, joints and ligaments. The muscles on both sides of the spine are automatically contacted when a person bends over and become relaxed when the person stands up. If the lumbar vertebrae are only controlled by the ligaments, and at the same time, improper force or external impact happens, an injury to the soft tissues may easily result. Because the lumbar nerves go into the lower limbs, an injury of the lumbar vertebrae may oppress and stimulate the lumbar nerves and will certainly give rise to pain, sensory disturbance and dyskinesia of the lower limbs. Lower back pain is therefore associated with leg pain. The causative factors for lumbocrural pain are many, among which trauma is a major factor. Lumbago is classified into acute traumatic lumbago and chronic lumbago. Chronic lumbocrural pain may appear with prolapse of the lumbar intervertebral disc (with partial sciatica) and lumbago due to kidney deficiency.

The lumbar spine is composed of five bones which are called vertebrae. Between the upper and lower vertebrae, there is an intervertebral disc (See Figs. 3-47/49), which is covered by fibrocartilage externally and internally contains soft, elastic and tremellose pulpiform nucleus. So the intervertebral disc bears the pressure and slows down the impulse between the vertebrae and help the movement of the spine in all directions. In movement the spine is able to change its shape. For example, when the spine is bent laterally, the pulpiform nucleus being oppressed on one side become thinner and those on the opposite side get thicker, and restore to their original when the spine is straightened. When the spine is bent forward, the pulpiform nucleus moves slightly, however, in case of sudden violence or heavy loadinng, or heavy force, the fibrous layer of the intervertebral disc may be ruptured and the pulpiform nucleus expand from the ruptured place and oppress the nerves. In the elderly, the symptoms are very significant because of degeneration of the intervertebral disc. From the top view of the cross section of the vertebrae, the shape of each vertebra looks like a jet plane (See Fig. 3-50). The connected pyramid and spinous process are called pedicle of the vertebral arch. The round hole in the centre is known as the vertebral foramen. When a series of vertebrae are connected, the vertebral foramen form a tubular structure named the vertebral canal, through which the spinal cord passes. Below the pedicle of the vertebral arch, there is a deep groove, which forms an oval hole with a shallow groove superior to the next vertebral arch. It is called an intervertebral foramen, where the spinal nerves pass through. In addition, there are some small joints which are named the superior and inferior articular process. The spinal cord passing through the vertebral canal is wrapped externally with a layer of periost known as the dura matter of the spinal cord. The nerves of the dura matter of the spinal cord are widely distributed and very sensitive. Once they are stimulated, pain results. The lumbar nerves originating from the spinal cord dominate the sense and movement of the lumbus, buttock, lower abdomen, vulva and lower limbs. After prolapse of the lumbar intervertebral disc, the pressure on the lumbar nerves will

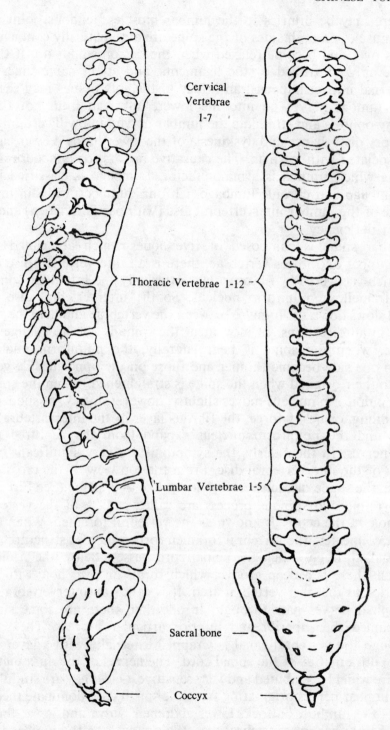

Cervical
Vertebrae
1-7

Thoracic Vertebrae 1-12

Lumbar Vertebrae 1-5

Sacral bone

Coccyx

Fig. 3-47

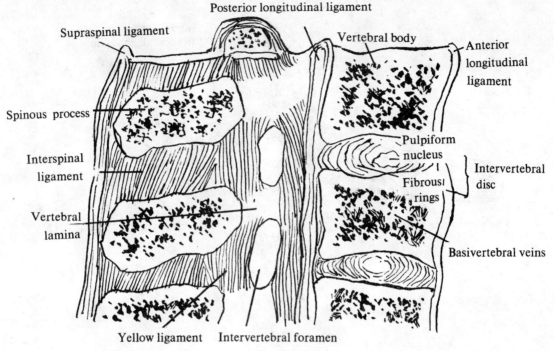

Fig. 3-48

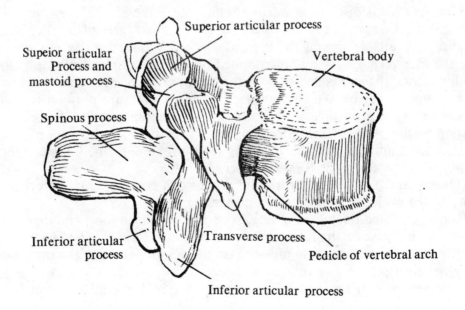

Fig. 3-49

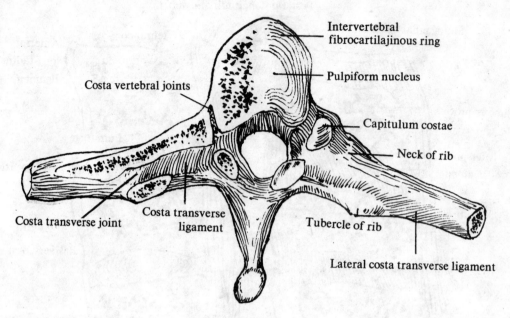

Fig. 3-50

give rise to lower back pain and leg pain.

The body is mostly supported by the lumbar spine, and weight supported gets heavier and heavier when going downward the spine. Therefore, prolapse of the lumbar intervertebral disc often occurs below the lumbus and there are many pathological conditions. In general, prolapse is directed posteriolaterally, because a clearance is available therewith. Prolapse in other directions is not common because the intervertebral disc is surrounded by the anterior and posterior longitudinal ligaments. If there is pressure on the dura matter of the spinal cord by the prolapse, simple lower back pain appears. If there is pressure only on the spinal nerves simple leg pain results. If the prolapse is large and there is pressure and stimulation on the intervertebral foramen, lower back pain and leg pain may occur simultaneously. Lumbocrural pain resulting from prolapse of the lumbar intervertebral disc is indicated by the following signs:

1) Intermittent pain (Better when the prolapse is contracted or absorbed and worse when the prolapse is out after contraction);

2) Pain aggravated during coughing, sneezing or defecation (The drop of the diaphram and increase of the intra-abdominal pressure promote the blood flow in the abdominal canal, increase the pressure on the spinal nerves or the dura matter of the spinal cord);

3) Disappearance of the physiological curvature of the lumbar vertebra (The contraction of the greater psoas muscle due to lower back pain may reduce the oppression of the prolapse posterior to the pyramid);

4) Pain aggravated in lowering the head and bending (Bending may increase the tensity, pressure and stimulation of the spinal nerve); and

5) Numbness at the lateral aspect of the lower limb or the leg without lower back pain and leg pain (The fifth spinal nerve is stimulated by the prolapse).

Lower back pain and leg pain are in direct ratio with the stimulation of the spinal cord or dura matter of the spinal cord by the prolapse. For instance, if the pressure and stimulation is heavier, the pain is more severe, (such as cutting, electric shock, burning and unbearable, but if the oppressing stimulation is light, only mild pain, numbness and soreness result.

2. Acute Traumatic Lumbago

Acute traumatic lumbago is a sudden pain due to trauma, such as improper carrying of heavy objects, traumatic injury, and external striking of the lumbus. Sometimes even coughing may cause acute lumbago.

Unilateral or bilateral severe pain, which is aggravated on exertion, makes forward and backward bending and left right rotation difficult. The patient was unable to roll over, and had a muscular spasm in the lower back, but showed no fracture and dislocation.

Treatment:

According to the findings in the examination, an acute lumbar sprain should be confirmed before the following manipulations are applied:

The patient is in a prone position with the back, lower back and buttock exposed.

1) Stroke the back and lower back 3-5 times in order to relax the non-injured tension of the muscle.

2) Grasp the Jianjing (G 21) point with the left and right hands, and then apply digital pressure with the thumb along the Bladder Meridian from Dazhu (B 11) to Baihuanshu (B 30), and from the Fufen (B 41) to the Zhibian (B 54) points. After digital pressing, stroking is followed with the same procedures on both the left and right sides. The strength exerted for the first digital pressing is light, that for the second time is heavy, and that for the third time is light again.

3) Press with the greater thenar of the palm from the Dazhu (B 11) to the Baihuanshu(B 30) points and from the Fufen (B 41) to the Zhibian (B 54) points from above to below three times. The strength exerted should be light, heavy and light. After one application of pressure to the points, slight stroking from above to below is followed.

4) Horizontally wipe in an opposite direction with the separating method from the lumbar fascia (i.e., from Shenshu, B 23 to Qihaishu, B 24) along the longitudinal axis of the lumbar muscle with the thumbs of both hands 5-7 times (See Fig. 3-51), then press the tender points towards the spinal vertebra with the thumb by means of the still pressing method (i.e., after pressing, keep still for a while).

5) Grasp the soft lumbus with the thumb and index finger of both hands (See Fig. 3-52), i.e., press the Jingmen (G 25) point with the thumb and the Zhangmen

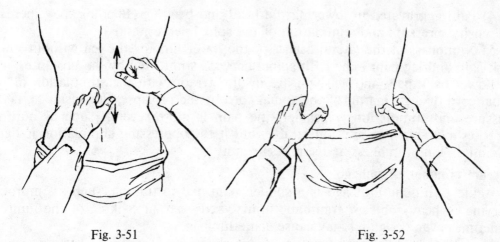

Fig. 3-51   Fig. 3-52

(Liv 13) point with the index finger. Repeatedly pick up and release for one minute to relax the muscle.

6) Pick up the Du Meridian from below to above with both hands and at the same time advance forward. Pick up the muscle of the point around the tenderness 3-5 times.

7) The thumbs of both hands are arranged in the form of "八", press first lightly and then heavily the points Shenshu (B 23), Qihaishu (B 24), Dachangshu (B 25), Guanyuanshu (B 26), Shangliao (B 31), Ciliao (B 32), Zhongliao (B 33), Xialiao (B 34) and Yaoyan (Extra) on both sides of the lumbar vertebrae. The time for pressing the significant tender points (such as Shenshu B 23, Qihaishu, B 24 and Yaoyangxue, Extra) may be longer, in combination with sedation, vibrating and concentric squeezing and pressing according to the requirements.

8) Horizontally push the posterior, medial and lateral sides of the left and right legs respectively from above to below with the palm, then press the Huantiao (G 30), Chengfu (B 36), Weizhong (B 40), Chengshan (B 57), Yinshi (S 33) and Fengshi (G 31) points with the thumb. Forcefully press the Kunlun (B 60) point with the nails of the thumb and index finger, percuss from the shoulder to the heel with the fist and the lateral palm, and apply slight strok before finishing the treatment.

The method for treating acute lumbago is called the method of treating the root cause by adult chiropractic, in which the wiping of the severe tender points at the lumbar region (i.e., Weishu, B 21, Sanjiaoshu, B 22 and Shenshu, B 23 points). It is a supplementary method for acute lumbar injury. Lumbago results from injury to the soft lumbar tissues, muscle spasm and stagnation of *qi* and blood. Severe pain is caused by the lumbar muscle synovium which is embedded on the lumbar vertebral small joint due to trauma, leading to the stimulation of the nervous fibres of the lumbar fascia and giving rise to local and general severe pain. The rigid and soft manipulations should be applied in order to relax the muscle and relieve the muscle spasm of the chest, back, lower back and the legs, thus regulating the circulation of *qi* and blood in the whole body. Some important Yang meridians and *Shu* points are located on the back and the patient cannot reach these points himself. Jianjing (G 21) is the main point connecting the meridians of the whole body. Therefore, grasping this point may activate the circulation of *qi* and blood. That's why grasping the Jianjing (G 21) point is frequently used. Prior to massage along the Bladder Meridian, grasp the Jianjing (G 21) point at least six times. At the same time, press from above to below and pick up the Shu points from below to above of the Du and the Bladder Meridians to regulate *qi* and blood of the five Zang and six Fu organs, so as to improve the disturbance of *qi* activity of the whole body resulting from an acute lumbar injury. The dialating-regulating method by wiping the embedded lumbar fascia and still-pressing method are applied to relax and loosen the contracted local fascia and to separate the small joint from the lumbar vertebra. Then the nerve fibre will no longer be stimulated, and the still-pressing method is thus able to relieve pain. In addition, heavy pressing of the points remote from the affected meridians on the lower back and leg may help to relieve lower back pain, because these points have the function to relieve lumbago and heavy pressure on these points may disperse the patient's attention so as to eliminate the "tender points" formed in the cerebral nerve centre.

Typical Case:

A male peasant aged 48 sprained his lower back when he was carrying a heavy load one day in 1972. The pain was so severe that the patient could not bend over backward. The condition was cured after being treated with the above-mentioned method for 3-6 minutes.

3. Prolapse of Lumbar Intervertebral Disc

Most cases of prolapse of the lumbar intervertebral disc are easily diagnosed according to the previously mentioned etiology. The simple diagnostic methods are as follows:

1) Straight leg raising test positive (not exceed 70°);

2) Deformity of scoliosis;

3) Tender point or rebound pain at the spinous process one cm lateral to the 3rd, 4th and 5th lumbar vertebrae and the 1st sacral vertebra;

4) Numb area on the leg; and

5) Weakness of the thumb dorsal extension (prolapse of the 4th and 5th lumbar intervertebral disc).

These five points can confirm the diagnosis of prolapse of the lumbar intervertebral disc. The direction of the prolapse is diagnosed by asking the patient to stand up with both hands placed at the lumbar region, and to rotate his body to the left and right sides. The prolapse is directed to the side on which pain apppears in combination with secondary sciatica. Refer to the comparison between the normal group and the abnormal group (See Figs. 3-53/54).

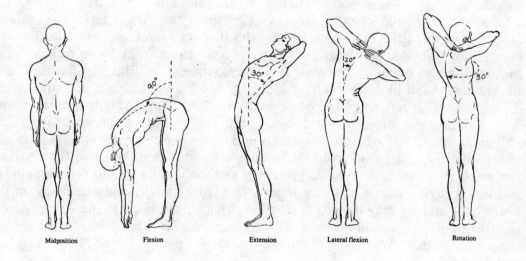

Midposition   Flexion   Extension   Lateral flexion   Rotation

Fig. 3-53

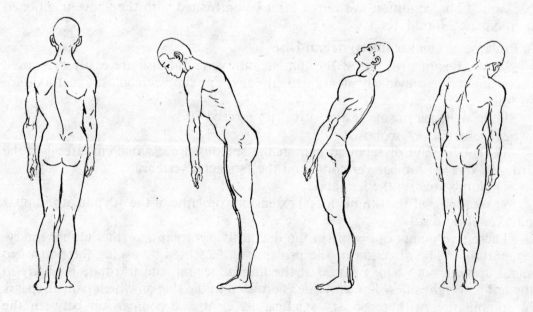

Fig. 3-54

Treatment:

1) The patient is in prone position and the doctor applies the adult chiropractic along the running course of the Bladder and Du Meridians on the back, lower back and buttock. For the detailed manipulations, refer to acute lower back pain, however, the procedures 4) and 5) are not necessary. After finishing the procedure, cover the back and lower back with clothes or a quilt to prevent the patient from catching cold.

2) Apply the following manipulations to the affected lower limb:

A. Horizontally push from the upper part of the Huantiao (G 30) point to the heel with the palm of one hand several times, and then laterally push the medial and lateral sides of the affected limb from above to below with the palms of both hands several times to activate the circulation of *qi* and blood in the lower limbs.

B. Tightly grasp the medial and lateral sides of the lower limbs from the ankle joint to the root of the thigh several times to dredge the meridians and collaterals, to relieve the muscle spasm and to promote blood reflux in the legs. Attention should be paid to the presence of a muscle spasm on the medial side of the thigh or to the appearance of marked pain during *tuina* treatment. If pain appears, grasp and knead, because a femoral adductor muscle spasm is also one of the causes of lower back pain.

C. Roll the posterior side of the affected limb several times, especially more on the popliteal fossa and sura.

D. Press the Huantiao (G 30), Chengfu (B 36), Yinmen (B 37), Weiyang (B 39), Chengjin (B 56), and Chengshan (N 57) points, and forcefully grasp the Kunlun (B 60) point on the affected side. In case of severe pain at the Huantiao (G 30) point, press with the fist tip or elbow tip instead of the thumb. In some patients, the muscles may twitch at Huantiao (G 30) and there may be general vibrating when pressing the Chengshan (B 57) point. In such a condition, slow pressure over a longer period of time on Huantiao (G 30) and Chengshan (B 57) may achieve better results. Then tap the posterior and both sides of the lower limb with the fist, palm and lateral palm, and lightly stroke twice before finishing the treatment. After that, the patient is in a supine position, push, roll and grasp the anterior side of the lower limb, press the Futu (S 32), Xuehai (Sp 10), Yanglingquan (G 34), Xuanzhong (G 39) and Fengshi (G 31) points with the thumb, then tap and percuss before finishing the treatment. In addition, the simplified procedures may be used on the healthy side to aid the recovery of the affected limb.

E. The patient is in a prone position and the doctor stands on the affected side of the patient, lifts the leg of the patient so that the knee is pulled up towards the chest and the doctor presses the affected limb for several minutes (See Fig. 3-45). Press Huantiao (G 30) and the nearby muscle with the thumb to seek the Ashi point. As soon as the tender point is found, press it with the thumb for a few minutes, or percuss it with the dorsum of the thumb. Pain can be greatly relieved.

F. For those who are unable to bend backward, not only the knee-to-chest-press (See Fig. 3-45) is applied for a few minutes, but also pressure on Huantiao (G 30) at the affected side is used. In case a marked tender point is found, percuss it with the fist tip several times. The pain can be satisfactorily relieved or eliminated.

G. For those who are unable to bend backward and have pain in bending the back-carrying method (See Fig. 2-35) may be applied to enhance the retroextention and to eliminate pain.

H. For those who are not suitable for the back-carrying method, but need traction, the holding maneuver (See Figs. 2-36/37) may be applied.

I. If the effect is not satisfactory after the treatment with the above-mentioned manipulations, massage of the chest and abdomen is combined. Knead and rub the abdomen for 10 minutes with both reinforcing and reducing, methods, then press the Daheng (Sp 15), Huangshu (K 16), Zhongshu (Du 7) and Guilai (S 29) points on the chest and abdomen with the thumb.

Typical Case:

An 18-year-old male student had lumbocrural pain for two years. The pain was increasingly aggravated and he couldn't hold heavy objects, do physical labour, sit or stand for a long time. He was treated by many therapies but without success. Examination: Anteflexion of the lower back 15°; lateral bending of the spine, right lateral back and costal prominence, lower back pain radiating to the leg, the test raising the leg straight of the affected side 25°, heel-buttock test positive. Diagnosis: prolapse of the lumbar intervertebral disc. Treatment: The above manipulations (A-E) were applied in the first treatment and an effect was obtained. The test raising the leg straight now showed 60°, anteflexion of the lower back was now 55°. The patient was treated once a day for more than half a month. The pain basically disappeared. All the tests were close to normal except for the lateral bending of the spine. The raising the leg straight test was 85°, the fingers could touch the ground in anteflexion. The patient could do some light work and the treatment stopped. The follow-up visits one year later showed him to be healthy.

4. Lower Back Pain Due to Kidney Deficiency

This condition results from internal injury. Traditional Chinese medicine holds that the lumbar region is where the kidney is housed and deficiency of the kidney may result in lower back pain, which is characterized by soreness and weakness of the lumbar region, vague pain, and free from the fixed pain. The pain is aggravated by physical labour done in a stooping position. The pain can be so severe as if the lumbus is broken. The stoop is not limited and primary organic disorders of the spine and soft tissues are absent. Excessive stooping will cause difficulty in straightening the back and straightening is possible with help from the hands. This problem may occur in any age group. This disease is accompanied by dizziness, tinnitus, insomnia and amnesia.

Treatment:

This disease may be treated by Chinese herbs which reinforce the kidney. *Tuina* therapy can achieve good results, in which the adult chiropractic is applied in combination with rubbing and pressing the lower back and kneading and palm-rubbing of the abdomen. The procedures are as follows:

1) Select the prone position and apply the adult chiropractic along the running course of the Bladder and Du Meridians. Each procedure is performed three times and increased to five times, mostly with the light and gentle reinforcing method. Rub the lumbus (horizontal rubbing and vertical rubbing alternately. Press, tap and percuss the Shenshu (B 23), Qihaishu (B 24), Dachangshu (B 25), Xiaochang-shu (B 27), Yaoshu (Du 2), Yaoyan (Extra), Mingmen (Du 4), Shangliao (B 31), Ciliao (B 32), Zhongliao (B 33) and Xialiao (B 34) points. The number of times should be increased according to the case.

2) Knead and rub the Qihai (Ren 6) and Guanyuan (Ren 4) points, poke and press the Futu (S 32), Xuehai (Sp 10), and Zusanli (S 36) points when the patient is in a supine position.

3) In case of dizziness and insomnia, *tuina* at the head is added, with emphasis on pressing, rubbing, pushing and kneading the Yintang (Extra 1), Zanzhu (B 2), Yuyao (Extra 3) and Sizhukong (SJ 23) points.

Typical Case:

A 34-year-old nurse came to the clinic in July 1978. Chief complaints: lower back pain as if broken, weakness of the legs, general lassitude, dizziness and insomnia for three years. She was treated by both Chinese and Western medications, but attacks still sometimes occurred. In recent days, the condition was aggravated. She rested at home for three months. Examination: No limitation of the functions, difficulty in straightening the back after stooping, no history of other problems. Two treatments were tried according to the methods for lower back pain due to kidney deficiency and neurosis. The patient felt comfortable, clear in mind and strong in the legs. After another six *tuina* treatments, the condition was improved, and the lower back pain greatly relieved. The patient could wash her hair and clothes with mild pain. The lumbar muscle was strengthened, the legs became strong, sleep improved and her appetite increased. Aftet twenty treatments the case was basically cured. The patient resumed her work, and no relapse was found in the follow-up visit half a year later.

5. Sequela of Fracture of the Coccyx

Lumbosacral pain resulted because a traumatic fracture of the coccyx did not heal. The patient was unable to sit and walk. Both Chinese and Western medication failed to achieve any effect. The patient has bed ridden for 7-8 months and recovered after *tuina* treatment.

Typical Case:

A woman aged 47 had terrible lumbosacral pain immediately after she fell down and hit her buttock on a hard object while she was carrying a heavy load. An X-ray showed a fractured coccyx. Treatment was given but without success. She was bed ridden for eight months. She had frequent pain and became emaciated.

She came to the clinic in April 1973. The adult chiropractic was applied to relieve the lower back pain, and the patient was advised to do exercises. After one course of treatment (14 treatments), the symptoms had basically disappeared. She could sit for a long time, walk and do some light housework. The follow-up visit two years later found no relapse.

6. Foot and Ankle Sprains:

This condition is due to contusion and sprain when jumping or falling down from a high place, which mostly injures the ligaments and fasciae. The trauma often occurs at the lateral side of the foot and ankle. Bruising, swelling, pain and impaired walking may appear. No fracture was found in an X-ray. *Tuina* may achieve immediate effects.

Treatment:

1) The patient sits in a bed or on a stool, while the doctor sits facing the patient. Put the affected foot on the doctor's knee.

A. Gently rub the foot several times to relax the foot, malleolus muscle and tendons and to relieve pain.

B. Hold the malleolus with one hand and treat the injured soft tissues at the malleolus and metatarsus with the thumb of the other hand, i.e., press and knead slightly from the affected malleolus to the toe and try to find out the marked pain in manipulation.

C. Knead, roll, press and rub the tender points and patiently knead and press the Jinmen (B 63) and Shenmai (B 62) points.

D. Knead and rub the ankle joint with the palms of both hands and at the same time shake it from left to right.

E. Grasp the bilateral Kunlun (B 60) point, press the tender point on the dorsum of the foot, pinch up both sides of the toes with one hand and wipe to the toes.

F. Hold the heel with one hand and gently shake and pull the toes with another hand.

G. Restore the abnormal malleolus tendons and the malpositioned bone seam with a skilled force, i.e., flex internally the affected limb, the patient holds the calf with both hands, the doctor supports the heel with one hand and holds the metatarsus from the lateral side with the other hand (See Figs. 3-55/56). Adduct the foot extremely several times and talk with the patient. When the patient is absent-minded and the foot is naturally relaxed, suddenly pull the extremely adducted foot anteriorinferiorly and a clicking sound is heard, suggesting that the technique has succeeded. Ask the patient to walk for a while and the pain is checked.

Typical Case

A college student aged 24 came to the clinic on July 2, 1981. His right foot was injured in a high jump match. Severe pain and swelling appeared at the external malleolus and the patient was unable to walk. Massage was applied for 15 minutes

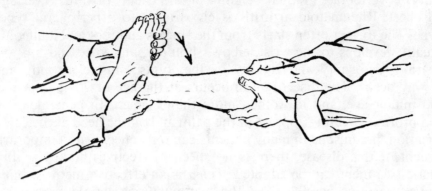

Fig. 3-55

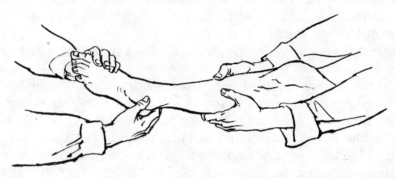

Fig. 3-56

according to the above-mentioned procedures. The swelling and pain disappeared and the patient could walk as usual. The next day he took part in the high jump match and won the championship. No relapse was found later.

X. RHEUMATOID ARTHRITIS

Rheumatoid arthritis, known as rheumatism of bone in traditional Chinese medicine, is a general chronic disease. Its etiology is still not clear so far, but cold-dampness is an important inducing factor. At the early stage, this disease has acute attacks and symmetrical and wandering joint swelling and severe pain. The disease attacks from the periost, cartilage, ligament, muscle tendon and then to the bone. The pathological change occurring in the spine is called spinal osteoarthritis, which mostly attacks from the sacroiliac articulation, and gradually spreads to the lower back, chest and neck, associated with hypertrophy and backward prominence of pyramid, calcification of anterior and posterior longitudinal ligaments, fusion and rigidity of vertebrae, gradual bending of the back, forward lowering of the head and chest. Rheumatoid arthritis is classified into a peripheral type and a central type. The former often starts from the fingers and foot and malleolus joints and gradually develops to the wrist, elbow, shoulder, and knee and hip joints. At a later period, deformity and rigidity of the joints, muscle atrophy and even crippling way occur. The disease often occurs at the age of 20-45, and mostly in youth and middle-age, and in women more than in men. In general, the pain is strong and profuse sweating appears in the palm and on the head at the early stage. The medication, prednisone in many patients can only check pain temporarily. For the treatment of this disease, there is no specific effective therapy so far. Only symptomatic treatment can be adopted. *Tuina* is an effective method, but should be applied as early as possible, and the manipulations should be accurate. No effects will be achieved for cases at an advanced stage of the disease.

Treatment

1. The doctor sits in front of the patient. Gentle stroking, twisting, kneading, pressing, grasping, stretching and flicking maneuvers are applied.

1) The operating sequence of the hand:

A. Before *tuina* is started, gently stroke the back of the hand and fingers several times.

B. Twist the swollen joints of the fingers, with more kneading and twisting on the large swollen joint. The time for twisting and kneading depends upon the pathological condition. More time twisting and kneading is needed in severe cases. Both sides of the finger joint should be kneaded and twisted up and down.

C. Press, knead, stretch and flick the fingers, i.e., based on the above mentioned method, press and knead the finger joints. The "general tendon" (at the midpoint of the wrist crease superior to the blood vessel) should be mostly pressed and kneaded. In case of failure in dispersing the tendons after pressing, kneading is required. After kneading for a while, pressing is followed in order to relax the tendons and muscles and activate the flow of *qi* and blood in the meridians. Subsequently, stretch the finger joint. By holding the upper interphalangeal articulation with one hand and the lower interphalangeal articulation with the other hand, slowly stretch the finger joint to separate the contractured ligament and the overlapped phalanx. If the separation tails push the finger joint back and stretch it again. When the separation occurs, a clicking sound is heard, and the dorsum of the finger becomes flat. The functions are now temporarily restored. If the separation is impossible, the stretching should not be forced in order to prevent injury of the ligaments. After stretching, flicking is advisable. The patient will feel pain and withdraw the hand in the process of flicking, but several flicks are required to separate the joints and to free the joint vessels.

D. Move the finger joint to see the flexion. Adduct the patient's wrist with one hand and pick up the Yangxi (LI 5) and Yanggu (SI 5) points with the thumb and middle finger of the other hand to loosen the wrist joint, and try to restore the adduction and backward flexion, then pick up the Hegu (LI 4) point and lightly stroke the hand before finishing the treatment.

2) Stroke, press, knead and roll the elbow and shoulder joints, emphasizing the pressing and keading of the Quze (P 3) and Chize (L 5) points, grasping of the Quchi (LI 11), Shaohai (H 3) and Shousanli (LI 10) points, and adduction and movement of the elbow joint. The treating method for the shoulder joint is similar to that for periarthritis of the shoulder, but simplified appropriately.

3) The treating method for the cervical joint is the simplified method for stiffneck.

2. The patient should be in a supine position and the doctor faces the patient and stands beside the bed. Apply the pushing, pressing, rolling and striking maneuvers at the hip, knee and malleolus joints and the lower limbs. The sequence is as follows:

1) Slightly stroke the lower limb with one hand and support the heel, hold the knee joint with the other hand to shake the hip joint. Flex the knee and ankle joints to see whether the motor functions are limited. Then perform the knee-to-chest test by keeping the knees as close as possible to the chest, and at the same time, pressure is added to flex the ankle and knee joints to 125°. This method relaxes the tendons and loosens the bones so as to move the knee and ankle joints. When there is pain, knead and press the painful region, especially the subcutaneous nodules and swelling. The patient should withstand the pressure and movement of the joints to prevent injury. The motor function should be enhanced without injury.

2) Press the Chongjie (Extra), Qichong (S 30), Biguan (S 31), Maibu (Extra), Xuehai (Sp 10), Futu (S 32), Sanyinjiao (Sp 6), Yinshi (S 33), Zusanli (S 36), Jiexi (S 41), Jinmen (B 63), and Shenmai (B 62) points. Grasping is used at the medial and lateral sides of the lower limb, while rolling is used at the anterior side of the lower limb.

3) Strike, percuss, beat and gently stroke the lower limb before finishing the treatment.

3. Take a supine position, carry out the heel-buttock test and add pressure. Press Huantiao (G 30) with the elbow tip, roll and strike the popliteal fossa, press (grasp) the Zhibian (B 54), Weizhong (B 40), Chengshan (B 57) and Kunlun (B 60) points, then percuss and slightly stroke with the fist. In case of headache and insomnia, a head massage is added. In case of a delicate constitution, chiropractic treatment is used, and in case of chest pain, pressing and rubbing the Tanzhong (Ren 17) point is added.

4. For spondylities, the routine chiropractic method is applied on the back and hand-overlapped pressing is added. (Ask the patient to breath deeply during pressing and strengthen the pressure when the bone joint is loosened.) If the spine is not rigid or bent, the back-carrying method may be used.

The above-mentioned manipulations are used alternately according to the pathological conditions.

Typical Case:

A female technician aged 35 came to the clinic in the spring in 1978. She was chilled by wind after sweating because of hyperkinesia ten years ago. She was treated in some hospitals in Shanghai, Suzhou and Beijing for about two years. The symptoms were controlled and relieved. In recent years, a relapse had occurred and the condition was gradually aggravated. She stopped the Western medication, but was treated by Chinese herbs and acupuncture for some time, and then by *tuina* therapy because of poor appetite. Examination: Pallor, dark circles, under the eyes, swollen fingers and inability to hold objects, wrist rigidity, impairment of the elbow and shoulder joints, pain and swelling of the ankle joints and the lower limbs, motor limitation of the knee and hip joints, inability to squat down, continuous pain, profuse sweating in the palms with the pain, poor appetite, pain aggravated at night, insomnia, some rigidity in the knee and ankle joints, clear bone crepitus in passive movement. After being treated with the above-mentioned manipulations, the patient generally felt comfortable, pain was relieved, joint movement improved, such as ability to grasp objects, and squatting down. After 5-6 *tuina* treatments, the condition gradually improved, the appetite increased and the patient slept sounder. Then the patient stopped the medication and continued *tuina* treatments for one month, and the effects were much better. The treatment was continued for another month. The swelling disappeared except for the ring finger, and the patient was able to grasp objects tightly, the wrist joint could be flexed, the patient could stand up quickly after squatting down, the stiffness in the knee and ankle joints improved, and the bone crepitus was reduced.

XI. GYNECOLOGICAL DISEASES

1. Dysmenorrhea

The symptoms of this condition are pain in the lower abdomen and lower back, and intolerable pain occurring a few days before or after menstruation. *Tuina* treatment of this condition often achieves good results.

Rubbing, kneading pushing and digital pressing are applied on the back and abdomen during the treatment, with emphasis on palm-rubbing and kneading on the abdomen and pushing and rubbing on the back. Gentle palm-rubbing and kneading are performed at the Guanyuan (Ren 4), Qihai (Ren 6), and Zhongji (Ren 3) points for 15 minutes in order to warm the meridians and to dispel cold, and slight and slow pushing and rubbing manipulated at the Shenshu (B 23), Mingmen (Du 4) and Gaohuang (B 43) points. The digital pressing should be frequently used and *tuina* should not be applied during menstruation.

Typical Case:

A 28-year-old worker came to the clinic on September 1, 1985, and complained of dysmenorrhea. During menstruation, distending pain in the lower abdomen and unsmooth menstrual flow occurred, which was diagnosed as dysmenorrhea due to stagnation of *qi*. Distending pain in the lower abdomen resulted from disturbance of *qi* activity and depression of the Chong and Ren Meridians. After being treated by *tuina* with the above-mentioned procedures five times, the distending pain was greatly relieved during the menstrual period, and the menstrual period lengthened from two days to four days. The *tuina* treatment was continued and the dysmenorrhea was cured. A few months later, the patient reported no more dysmenorrhea and now had regular menstrual periods.

2. Mastitis

This condition is ascribed either to internal retention of milk leading to distending pain, or to disturbed secretion of milk giving rise to mammary swelling, distension and pain for during lactation or after an abortion. At the initial stage, *tuina* therapy often achieves good results. However, any breast abscess should be treated by surgery.

Gentle grasping is applied in combination with kneading. Tap slightly the shoulders, back and the affected breast with the first four fingers. Main points: Tap gently and rhythmically to vibrate the breasts somewhat without pain. Tap for a longer time, then support the breast with one hand, push and knead the breast gently with the other hand. Pushing the breast is different from that of a large area on the body surface. The manipulation should be light and free from squeezing. Either by supporting the breast (from the nipple to the chest) or slightly holding the breast with one hand, stroke and gently push from the root of the breast to the nipple with the other hand to disperse the stagnation, then apply pressure at the Rugen (S 18) point with the middle finger, and pressing at the Tianxi (Sp 18), Ximen (P 4), Jianjing (G 21), Zulinqi (G 41) and Dushu (B 16) points. Finally, standing behind the patient, the doctor pushes the hypochondrium with both hands from the subaxillary region obliquely to the costal region several times.

Typical Case:

A worker aged 29 came to the clinic on July 11, 1978. Chief complaints: ulceration, pain and swelling of the nipple, and cacogalactia because the baby liked to bite the nipple during lactation. She had distension, fullness, expansion and pain and medium hard nodules in the breast. Since the medication achieved only slow effects, the patient asked to have *tuina* treatment. The routine method for mastitis was followed with gentle kneading and pushing for 40 minutes. The patient felt relaxed and the pain was greatly relieved. After being treated continuously for three days, the case was completely cured.

3. Climacteric Syndrome

The changes that occur during menopause may cause some symptoms such as anemia, endocrine disturbances, an abnormal menstrual period, tidal fever, palpitation, lassitude, insomnia and irritability may appear. *Tuina* is effective in this case, but should be performed before and after menstruation.

1) The routine chiropractic method is applied on the back when the patient is

in a supine position.

2) The routine *tuina* methods used on the abdomen are mainly kneading and palm-rubbing when the patient is in a prone position.

3) Routine massage is performed on the head when the patient is in a sitting position. (Reducing for excess syndrome and reinforcing for a deficiency syndrome).

Typical Case:

A 50-year-old cadre came to the clinic in 1985. Chief complaints: dizziness, insomnia, lassitude, irritability and lower back pain for about one year. Medication failed to have any effect. Normal nourishment, shallow complexion, deep and string-taut pulse and anemia for half a year. Diagnosis: Menopause. After being treated intermittently 17 times with the above mentioned procedures, with the emphasis on reinforcing, the dizziness, lassitude and insomnia were greatly relieved. Medication was taken to strengthen the effect because the patient had busy housework.

XII. MISCELLANEOUS DISEASES

1. Obesity

Obesity is a disease of excessive accumulation of body fat resulting from the intake of too many calories. In general, weight exceeding the normal body weight by 20% is obesity. An endocrine dysfunction of the nervous system may reduce the regulating ability of the movement, ingestion, and metabolism, as a result of obesity. In addition, obesity is also related to hypokinesia and inheritance. For obesity, the excessive accumulation of fat is present not only in the subcutaneous tissues, but also in the abdominal cavity (such as in the greater omentum, kidney, heart periphery and myocardium). Therefore, obesity is often associated with chronic visceral diseases, such as asthma, cardiectasis, constipation and hyposexuality. For obese patients, *tuina* therapy may achieve good results in addition to some appropriate movements (such as slow running).

Treatment:

Tuina is mainly performed on the abdomen and the four limbs, with emphasis on pushing, grasping and rolling.

1) Palm-rubbing, rolling, picking up, grasping, separating, joining, slight tapping and puncturing are performed on the abdomen for 10 minutes each to promote intestinal peristalsis and contraction of the abdominal muscle. In this way, some fat is consumed after being transformed into heat, thus the accumulation of body fat is reduced.

2) Apply *tuina* on the four limbs, with emphasis on pushing, grasping and rolling. The procedures are basically similar to those introduced before. Tight grasping of the muscles of the arms is mostly done, while pushing and rolling are used less and pushing the leg muscles is frequently applied. Progressive grasping

of both sides of the thigh and leg is mostly done (See Fig. 3-40), while pushing (from above to below) and rolling are often used at the anterior and posterior sides. Tapping, percussion and thumb-pressing of the points at the fat place are done, and more frequently at the back side. In a word, the method is the same as mentioned before, but it is somewhat prolonged in order to increase the opening quantity of the muscular capillaries (increased several times than before the treatment), thus the muscle metabolism is improved, the consumption of fat increased and the purpose of reducing the weight achieved.

3) Pushing, pressing and grasping on the chest, back and lower back as the procedures mentioned before. After *tuina* treatment, the patient will feel light. The patient is advised to do physical exercise in order to further reduce of the weight.

2. Constipation

The infrequent evacuation of dry feces with no bowel movement in more than 48 hours is regarded as constipation, which is clinically classified into heat constipation, *qi* constipation, deficiency constipation and cold constipation. Heat constipation results either from the excessive intake of hot food, leading to accumulation of heat in the intestines and stomach and burning of the fluids, causing dryness in the intestinal tract, or from heat retained after a febrile disease at the later period, leading to the consumption of body fluids. *Qi* constipation is usually due to disturbance of *qi* flow and dysfunction of *qi* transportation and transformation caused by anxiety, anger or emotional frustration. Constipation of the deficiency type appears after disease or delivery, and in the elderly with deficiency of both *qi* and blood. Deficiency of *qi* will cause weakness of the transportation of the large intestines and deficiency of blood will fail to moisten the intestines. Cold constipation is caused by excessive Yin-cold in the elderly and a delicate constitution obstructing Yang *qi*.

Treatment:

1) *Tuina* is performed on the abdomen when the patient is in a prone position. Palm-rub along or against several times from the upper abdomen to the umbilicus and then around it. If a hard substance is felt by the palm in the abdominal cavity, the rubbing should be done slowly and gently for a longer time. After the intra-abdominal hardness becomes softer, the rubbing may be carried out a little faster. Then undertake rubbing around the umbilicus with the palms several times, and advance forward during rubbing with the palm from above to below, push divergently from the umbilicus with the forehand and then jointly to the umbilicus. Rub transversely above the transverse line of the umbilicus, roll and knead slightly in a large circle along the running course of the ascending and descending colons on the left and right sides of the lumbar region, then gently percuss with the lateral palm and slightly stroke with the palms of both hands several times before finishing the treatment. The manipulations should be kept slow and gentle gradually increasing the strength. The purpose is to strengthen the intestinal peristalsis and to moisten the fluids of the intestinal wall and to promote fecal discharge.

2) Strongly press and grasp the important points with three fingers, press the medial side of the left costal region at Daheng (Sp 15), bilateral Tianshu (S 25), Wushu (G 27), and the midpoint of the groin, and then grasp the left and right soft lumbus with both hands.

3) Press and knead the left and right Weicang (B 50) and Huangmen (B 51) points with the thumbs of both hands when the patient is in a supine position, and push straight downward from the Weicang (B 50) to the Zhibian (B 54) points from slow to fast several times.

4) Hot food and physical exercise and walking after meals should be encouraged.

3. Incontinence of Urine

Incontinence of urine refers to the inability to control urination and most problems are of the deficiency syndrome. This condition is ascribed to insufficiency of primary kidney *qi* and deficiency-cold in the lower *jiao*. For instance, frequent urination with profuse, clear white urine is due to deficiency of kidney Yang leading to failure in controlling water, so the treatment is directed to warm and reinforce the kidney Yang; while frequent and rapid urination with scanty and dark yellow urine is due to Yin deficiency and the presence of heat. Frequent and urgent urination with scanty urine associated with abdominal distension is due to depression of liver *qi*, and frequent and rapid urination with urine like grease and great thirst is regarded as diabetes.

Treatment:

1) Gently and slowly knead around the umbilicus and the lower abdomen clockwise with the palms of both hands when the patient is in a supine position with the knees adducted.

2) Rub to and fro horizontally at the lumbar region when the patient is in a prone position with the palm of one hand, and then push horizontally from the Changqiang (Du 1), Yaoshu (D 2) to Shenshu (B 23) points downward to upward until the skin region becomes warm.

3) Digitally press the Qihai (Ren 6) and Guanyuan (Ren 4) points for 30 minutes.

Typical Case

Two female cadres aged 59 and 60 had the similar symptoms, such as frequent, rapid and urgent urination with scanty urine, enuresis in the last couple of years, ability to control the urine out of the house, but failure in controlling it at home. Having been treated with the above-mentioned method 5-7 times, the disease was cured.

4. Arteriosclerotic Senility

Arteriosclerotic senility, a general arteriosclerosis associated with old age, is characterized by sclerosis of the aorta, cerebral arteries, renal artery and conducting arteries and medium-sized arteries of the four limbs. The typical characteristics include chronic disease, multiple disease, being bed-ridden longterm, deficiency of *qi* and disinclination to speak, heaviness of the head, difficulty sitting, difficulty walking without the help of a cane, failure in walking, inability to hold objects and inability to manage the daily life, paraplegia and dementia. Medication did not help the condition much but *tuina* therapy achieved better effects.

Treatment:

With gentle manipulations *tuina* therapy is applied to the whole body. The manipulations are the same as those mentioned before, mainly light, slow and gentle. For fat patients, forceful manipulations may be used, but care should be taken to prevent fractures.

Typical Cases:

A female cadre aged 79 suffered from several kinds of internal diseases. She was so weak that she could not walk without help. After being treated with *tuina* therapy for a short time, her vitality increased and she gradually recovered. In addition to some symptoms of pulmonary heart disease, gastrointestinal disease, insomnia, lumbocrural pain, and neurosis were all relieved. She could get up early in the morning and go for a walk in the courtyard and in the nearby park.

A veteran doctor aged 82 had paraplegia after windstroke for two years. He had to lie in bed and could not turn over, sit and walk, associated with dementia. After being treated with *tuina* therapy several times, he could turn over, sit down and walk for a few steps with the help of stick. The treatment was continued for another several times, and his vitality increased so he could talk and sing.

5. Tympanites Due to Stagnation of *Qi*

This condition refers to abnormal distention due to the presence of air in the abdomen and chest, with tight stretching of the skin, sound audible by percussion or large abdomen with thickening of skin. It mostly results from stagnation of *qi*.

Treatment:

1) Massage the chest and abdomen for 10 minutes using the same manipulations as for hemiplegia.

2) Massage the Bladder Meridian and Du Meridian on the back for 10 minutes with the same manipulations as for insomnia. The difference is to use the forearm and the elbow tip to press and knead the back in order to soften the stagnated and thickened muscles.

3) Digitally press the Xuanji (Ren 21), Tanzhong (Ren 17), Jingmen (G 25) and Qihai (Ren 6) points.

Typical Case:

A female worker aged 51 came to the clinic on September 10, 1986. Chief complaints: abdominal distention for about 20 years, associated with the feeling of *qi* rushing upward, distending pain and poor appetite. She had been treated many times but with no response. She was examined many times and nothing could be found. She was obese and her abdomen measured 105 cm. Diagnosis: tympanites due to stagnation of *qi*. After being treated with the above-mentioned method for six times, the circumference of the abdomen was reduced by 15 cm. Another seven treatments were administered and the abdominal distention disappeared. The treatment was therefore completed and pills for strengthening the spleen were taken to consolidate the effects.

中国推拿疗法

王 甫 编著

*

ⓒ外文出版社

（中国北京百万庄路 24 号）

邮政编码 100037

北京外文印刷厂印刷

中国国际图书贸易总公司发行

（中国北京车公庄西路 35 号）

北京邮政信箱第 399 号　邮政编码 100044

1994 年(16 开)第一版

（英）

ISBN 7 - 119 - 01674 - 1 /R·107(外)

04860

14 - E - 2505S